GLIADIN

SOD
GLIADIN

THE
ULTIMATE DEFENSE
AGAINST DISEASE
AND AGING

CARL GERMANO,
R.D., C.N.S., L.D.N.

TWINS STREAMS
KENSINGTON PUBLISHING CORP.
http://www.kensingtonbooks.com

TWIN STREAM BOOKS are published by

Kensington Publishing Corp.
850 Third Avenue
New York, NY 10022

First Kensington Paperback Printing: October 2001
10 9 8 7 6 5 4 3 2 1

Printed in the United States of America

ACKNOWLEDGMENT

I wish to extend my sincere appreciation to Bernard Dugas, Ph.D., Janice Kane, D.O., and Lisa Turner for their contributions to this book.

CONTENTS

INTRODUCTION

The population of the United States is rapidly aging, and Americans are living longer than ever before. Life expectancy is now almost 80 years—a big difference from the 49-year estimate in 1900. Currently, almost one-third of the annual U.S. health care expenditure, $300 billion, is attributed to older Americans. These individuals suffer from a number of pre-disease conditions and chronic diseases such as arthritis, hypertension, cardiovascular disease, cancer, diabetes, immune deficiency, memory and cognitive impairment, and depression. These conditions are constant and lifelong ailments. There is a great demand among these people for products that enhance the quality of life. In addition, most of these aging individuals have seen their parents die from similar illnesses and are determined to do what they can to reduce their own risk and ease their minds by defending against the onset and progression of these conditions. Today, one dietary ingredient stands out as the most important disease defender by virtue of the fact that each and every cell in the body manufactures it and depends upon its existence to survive and to prevent disease and aging: superoxide dismutase, also known as SOD.

What Is Superoxide Dismutase?

As we go about our lives, we never stop and think about what a monumental achievement it is for our bodies to last as long as they do. Compare the human body to a car, which has an average life span of 10 to 15 years—if it's well maintained. What if that same car ran continuously for 60, 70, 80, or even 90 years and had the ability to maintain itself? All you had to do was get in, add some fuel, and turn the key! Unlike the automobile, we survive internal and external assaults to the body because of a process called homeostasis, the ability of the body to maintain a state of equilibrium in the face of internal and external variations or stressors such as pollution, bad food, and emotional and physical stress. Homeostasis affords us a long life because the body is able to control most conditions that are potentially detrimental. Without these processes, our life span would be less than that of a well-maintained car. One of the most important control mechanisms is our body's ability to maintain an oxidant/antioxidant balance.

The body produces potentially damaging oxygen free radicals on a daily basis. It is an inevitable process, a by-product of energy metabolism, diet, and environmental influences. The body also produces free radicals as a defense against viruses and bacteria. Infected cells, as well as the immune system, produce free radicals to inactivate and destroy invading microbes. Under normal conditions, the deluge of free radicals is usually eliminated by antioxidants. However, as we age and are exposed to disease and other stressors, excess free radicals and lower cellular defenses can cause inflammation, cellular tissue toxicity, degenerative diseases, and accelerated aging.

Researchers speculate that free radicals may play a role in the aging process, as evidenced by increased levels of free radicals and accumulated free radical tissue damage in aging animals. The free radical theory states that aging is the result of imperfect protection against tissue damage resulting from free radicals and that this damage ultimately leads to our demise. More than 15 years of research has specifically focused on SOD's relationship to aging. The evidence for humans, however, requires further research. Even though SOD supplementation has been shown to increase the life span of simpler life forms, such as mosquitoes and worms, well-designed studies on humans are necessary. Interestingly, associations between aging and SOD levels in the body are inconsistent because certain older individuals seem to have higher levels of SOD than their younger counterparts. Some researchers have speculated that it may not be the amount of SOD in the body that plays a part in the aging process, but rather the body's ability to quickly produce higher levels of SOD during times of increased oxidative stress. Think of it as the response time of an ambulance to a call. The longer it takes for that ambulance to answer the call, the greater the risk to the person in need. Older individuals' SOD response time to increased oxidative stress is lower than that of younger individuals. Older individuals with a higher SOD response time than the norm live longer, suggesting that the preservation of this response time correlates with longevity. Because aging is poorly understood and under-researched at the molecular level, further studies need to be done to accurately associate free radicals with aging and, more importantly, to verify that supplementing with antioxidants can enhance longevity. The process of aging is a highly complex interaction between the body's genetic, environmental, and internal synergies and its antioxidant system. However, the implication that free radicals play a role in the aging process is a testament to their powerful influence on health.

Free Radicals

What are free radicals and how can something so small cause so much damage? The atom is the most basic unit of matter; it makes up everything in our body. Atoms combine to form molecules such as proteins, fats, and carbohydrates. The typical atom has a nucleus, which contains positively charged particles called protons. Orbiting the nucleus like planets around a star are negatively charged particles called electrons. For an atom to be stable, it must contain the same number of protons and electrons, so that the charges are balanced. However, through normal metabolic processes and from external toxins such as cigarette smoke, alcohol, bad food, air pollution, and radiation, an atom may lose or gain an electron. Because an atom must have an equal number of electrons and protons, losing or gaining an electron results in an atom that is unstable and highly reactive—a free radical.

To become stable, a free radical attacks another atom or molecule and steals or adds an electron. This is where our problems begin, because in the process of stabilizing the first free radical, another is created, and this reaction will continue with each subsequent free radical creating another free radical. In other words, it sets off a chain reaction. Free radicals are indiscriminate assailants, attacking important molecules such as carbohydrates, proteins, and fats (parts of each and every cell of the body) and altering their intended function. These dysfunctional molecules can impair normal metabolism. Fats, for example, are the key component of cell membranes and play important roles in cellular metabolism. Free radicals that damage cellular membranes alter normal cell metabolism, and if a significant number of cells are damaged, you have the beginning of a disease. Perhaps the most critical component of our body that is susceptible to free radical attack is the very blueprint of our genetic existence: deoxyribonucleic acid (DNA). It is estimated that free radicals attack DNA approximately 100,000 times *per cell* each day. We will see in a later chapter what implications damaged DNA has on our health and why it is important to quench free radical chain reactions before they have a chance to damage our cells.

We can see that it is not the individual free radical that causes disease. The damage caused by a single free radical is minute. Rather, it is the total effect of countless numbers of free radicals produced in the body that causes a deterioration of health. In a healthy person, antioxidant nutrients and enzymes buffer free radicals. When this delicate balance between oxidant and antioxidant molecules is upset, various inflammatory and degenerative conditions can appear. Therefore, if free radicals are the impetus behind disease, it is logical to assume that diet may delay or even prevent disease processes. The idea that diet plays a role in the oxidant/antioxidant balance is enhanced because of the biological role many essential nutrients, such as vitamins C and E, play in the prevention of free radical production and resultant disease. In addition to antioxidants consumed as food, a number of antioxidant enzymes are manufactured within the body and serve as a frontline defense against free radicals. Enzymes are protein-based substances found in every cell of all living animals and plants that initiate or assist chemical reactions. One of the most important antioxidant enzymes is superoxide dismutase. SOD is truly the cell's master defense mechanism to quench free radicals and prevent disease.

Superoxide dismutase has been of interest to medical professionals since its discovery in 1968. It was first used in an injectable form to treat arthritis in adults and breathing problems in infants and to serve as a companion therapy to cancer treatment. A mutase is a type of enzyme that initiates the rearrangement of atoms in a molecule, and SOD's primary function is to convert the free radical superoxide (O_2^-) into hydrogen peroxide (H_2O_2), a less harmful free radical. Among the free radicals, superoxide is the most powerful and dangerous. This is because, due to its chemical structure, it requires three electrons to rebalance itself. When it snatches those three electrons from other molecules, it creates even more imbalance than a conventional free radical looking for only one electron. Also it tends to rebalance itself more rapidly, creating more superoxides, with the potential to cause a lot more damage. A reactive oxygen species (ROS) free radical, it has been associated with all kinds of degenerative processes, including arthritis, cancer, Alzheimer's disease, and Parkinson's disease. Additionally, superoxide along with nitric oxide leads to the generation of peroxynitrite, which is principally responsible for the death of the cell. Because superoxide is so potentially damaging, SOD exists in two forms in the cell. In the mitochondria, which are the energy-producing structures of the cell, SOD is present as a manganese-containing enzyme. In the cytoplasm of the cell, copper and zinc are the primary metals found in the structure of SOD. The presence of SOD in both the mitochondria and the cytoplasm ensures that much of the superoxide is converted to hydrogen peroxide. In later chapters, we will see what happens when superoxide is allowed to run rampant in the body and how SOD can help delay and, in some cases, prevent the disease process.

This book examines the correlation between SOD and disease prevention and treatment and the issues surrounding injectable bovine sources of SOD versus pervious and newly developed oral forms of vegetarian SOD. While in the past injectable SOD from bovine sources was used, today we have SOD/gliadin: the first orally available, vegetarian source of SOD and a revolutionary breakthrough in nutraceutical development. Maybe you or someone you know is suffering from cancer, heart disease, or some other malady. Each chapter answers the very imortant questions, "why supplement with the master cellular defense enzyme SOD?" and "Why go through the trouble of producing an oral supplement of SOD?"

CHAPTER 1

SOD AND ARTHRITIS

Not just a minor inconvenience or moderately painful condition, arthritis is serious business. Its effects can be so devastating that it is considered the number-one cause of disability in the United States. Arthritis is a chronic, debilitating condition that causes severe pain, inflammation, and disability of the joints. Nearly 40 million Americans suffer from arthritis or joint pain. And as the Baby Boomers age, arthritis continues to become more widespread. By the year 2020, it is estimated, arthritis will affect nearly 60 million Americans.

To date, research has supposed genetics, hormonal imbalances, and environmental factors to be responsible for this condition, though the exact cause is unknown. A myriad of medications and treatments for arthritis, including surgery, joint replacement, and prescription drugs, are available. Arthritis is most commonly treated with steroidal drugs such as cortisone; nonsteroidal anti-inflammatory drugs (NSAIDs) including aspirin, naprosyn, and ibuprofen; and the new "super aspirins" COX-2 inhibitors. The problem with most over-the-counter and prescription pain medications lies not in their use but in their overuse. Many people feel they cannot live without them. Statistics show that the vast majority of the human population uses over-the-counter pain drugs on a regular basis. Why is this so bad? Because these drugs have unpleasant to dangerous side effects, including nausea, stomach irritation, stomach and duodenal ulcers, and kidney and liver damage. By reducing the inflammation associated with arthritis, SOD/gliadin can offer a safe and effective alternative with no side effects.

Types of Arthritis

Defined as the inflammation of a joint, "arthritis" is a general term for progressive joint disease marked by pain and stiffness. There are nearly 100 different forms. The most prevalent and painful are osteoarthritis (OA), rheumatoid arthritis (RA), and arthritis associated with systemic lupus erythematosus.

- **Osteoarthritis,** characterized by erosion of the articulations between bones, is the most common form and is generally associated with aging. It generally attacks individual joints, usually those that bear weight, such as the feet, knees, hips, and spine. It results in chronic pain and low-grade inflammation.

• **Rheumatoid arthritis** is an autoimmune disease. It is painful and crippling, causing inflammation and destruction of joints throughout the body.

• **Ankylosing spondylitis,** similar to rheumatoid arthritis, is a disease of the spine, marked by pain and stiffness that may progress until the spine is rigid. It attacks men ten times as often as women.

• **Gout** usually begins in the joints of the big toe. It is caused by excess uric acid, which forms painful crystals in the joints that result in pain and inflammation.

• **Bursitis,** an inflammation of the bursa (such as in tennis elbow), causes inflammation, pain, and swelling.

• **Juvenile arthritis** causes swelling of the lymph nodes and spleen, rashes, and retarded growth. It occurs in children, sometimes beginning in infancy, and is similar to rheumatoid arthritis.

• **Systemic lupus erythematosus** (lupus) is a connective tissue disease that affects the joints as well as the skin and internal organs. It generally strikes women between 20 and 40 years old.

Rheumatoid arthritis differs from other forms of arthritis because of the way it occurs in the body. Rheumatoid arthritis is an autoimmune disorder. That means the body's immune system literally begins to attack itself at the area of the joints and connective tissues. It is thought that monocytes (white blood cells) gone awry are in part responsible for arthritis. Monocytes are one of the body's primary defenders against foreign invaders. When pathogens attack the body, the immune system calls forth an army of defender and scavenger white blood cells. Lymphocytes identify the intruders, and phagocytes surround and digest them. Monocytes scavenge dead cells and debris at the site of an infection or injury. For reasons yet unknown, monocytes sometimes run amok, turning into macrophages and releasing inflammatory material into surrounding tissue. This triggers additional lymphocytes and monocytes to be called to the area, where they are then attacked. The inflammatory mass grows and begins to destroy bone and cartilage. The result is joint erosion and, ultimately, destruction.

Arthritis, Inflammation, and SOD

All forms of arthritis include inflammation as the root of the pain. And inflammation has been linked to oxidative stress in numerous scientific studies. Just like the lung of the asthmatic, the joints of the arthritic are caught in a vicious circle of free radical production, swelling, and cellular damage. The typical chain reaction looks like this: Phagocytosing cells, or immune system cells (such as white blood cells and macrophages) that consume foreign invaders (such as bacteria and cell debris) produce ample amounts of the ROS free radical superoxide. Superoxide is one of the weapons they use to destroy foreign invaders. But when superoxide is produced in excess, it begins to destroy surrounding cell tissue including sensitive joint tissues such as the cartilage and the synovial membrane, which secretes the synovial fluid that lubricates the joints. Once damaged, these tissues deteriorate and swell, eliciting a further immune response, which sends phagocytes to the area to consume the debris, starting the cycle over again.

In the case of osteoarthritis, this type of oxidative stress may be externally stimulated through injury or other causes. In rheumatoid arthritis, the out-of-control immune system perpetuates the damage. In both cases, however, the damage to the joint tissue can be alleviated and slowed by counteracting the production of superoxide with SOD/gliadin, the first orally bioavailable, vegetarian form of supplemental SOD.

What the Studies Show

A number of scientific studies point to SOD as a valuable treatment for arthritis. Free radical—

specifically superoxide—damage in the joint tissue appears to be a primary cause of arthritis. By quenching free radicals, SOD can slow the development and progression, and may actually prevent the onset, of certain kinds of arthritis. And unlike steroids and other medications commonly used to treat arthritis, SOD/gliadin has no side effects and is safe to use, as compared to the bovine injectable forms used in most studies. Yes, it is true that the studies used injectable SOD at the site of injury. It may very well be possible that an oral form of SOD may play an important role in recovery. SOD/gliadin is the first orally available vegetarian form of this critically important enzyme.

- **SOD reduces free radicals in joint tissue.** A study tested orgotein on patients with RA or OA. "Orgotein" is the generic name for copper-zinc superoxide dismutase. They found that injections three times per week in patients with RA induced significant improvement within 3 months. OA patients received one injection a week for 8 weeks and also showed marked improvement. The relief from the arthritis is presumed to be in the reducing action of the SOD on free radicals, specifically superoxide, in the joint tissue. This can slow down or arrest the cycle of inflammation and free radical production.

- **Free radicals damage joints.** Another study, in *Revista do Hospital das Clinicas; Faculdade de*

Medicina Da Universidade de São Paulo, also associated free radicals with progression of RA. The study supports the idea that free radicals contribute to the damage in joints found in RA. By reducing the level of free radicals, SOD can slow the development and progression of RA.

• **Free radicals cause inflammation in joints.** A study in *Immunology Today* suggests that oxidative stress contributes to the progression of inflammation into chronic diseases such as RA and other inflammatory disorders. The researchers found that damage from free radicals at the point of inflammation can cause permanent genetic changes that may lead to chronic conditions. By fighting free radicals, SOD may halt the development of RA.

• **Free radicals stimulate the damaging effects of the immune system in joint tissue.** A study in the *British Medical Bulletin* describes the mechanical process of how free radicals are produced in RA joints. Normal, healthy joints move freely and get plenty of circulation. But in RA, the joint cavity pressure is raised by the inflammation to the degree that normal movement can actually collapse capillaries and small blood vessels. This leads to an injury called hypoxia, or lack of oxygen to the tissue. Research has shown that hypoxia induces ROS free radical production. This production of additional free radicals in turn stimulates an immune response, exacerbating and repeating the damage. It would appear that reducing the level of free radicals would be the easiest way to break the inflammatory vicious cycle responsible for damaging the joints. Supplementation with antioxidants such as SOD/gliadin might be one way to break the cycle.

• **Antioxidants such as SOD provide protection from RA.** A study in *Annals of Rheumatoid Disease* supports the theory that ROS free radicals create tissue damage in RA, and that antioxidants can provide protection from RA. The study included more than 1,400 patients and their follow-ups over a 20-year period. The conclusions found a significant association between low antioxidant levels and the risk of developing RA. This suggests that free radical–quenching antioxidants actually prevent the onset of RA.

• **SOD suppresses inflammation in RA.** A study in *Free Radical Research Communications* examined the effect of SOD on a variety of disorders including RA. In this study, RA patients were given injections twice a week for 8 weeks. Patients with severe RA—including deformities of the joints, intense pain and swelling, restriction of movement, and posture changes—showed dramatic improvements following the treatment. In particular, one female patient arrived at the hospital in a wheelchair, unable to walk because of RA. After 8 weeks of treatment, she was walking on crutches, and soon after, she could walk unaided. The results of the study show SOD to be an inflammatory suppressant and preventative. Also, the researchers note traditional therapies for RA can have many side effects, whereas SOD is not only efficient but also nontoxic in the body.

• **SOD may be a therapeutic agent in RA.** A study in *Biochimica and Biophysica Acta* was designed specifically to test the efficiency of liposomal SOD. The liposomal form of SOD is encased in a substance to protect it from breaking down too quickly in the body. Researchers found that liposomal SOD helped target specific areas, such as the joints, in the treatment of RA. Their study was based upon previous evidence that free radicals and oxidative stress are contributors to the RA condition. They said that SOD may be used as a therapeutic agent in the treatment of RA.

• **SOD provides long-term relief.** A study in *Scandinavian Journal of Rheumatology* found that treatment of OA with orgotein gave long-term relief to patients. This double-blind study included 36 patients and compared treatment with orgotein (SOD) to treatment with methylprednisolone acetate, a steroidal anti-inflammatory. The treatment consisted of one injection every other week for 6 weeks and a 6-month follow-up. The long-term improvements were significantly better with the use of orgotein. And although there was a mild reaction with the injection of the orgotein including some swelling, warmth, and pain, it spontaneously disappeared within days. Also, orgotein doesn't cause some of the side effects found with injectable steroids such as methylprednisolone acetate, including joint infection, muscle wasting, tendon rupture, and skin atrophy.

• **SOD significantly reduces joint damage in RA.** One open clinical study published in *Therapie* used liposomal bovine injectable SOD to treat patients with severe RA. The drug was administered twice a week for 3 months and was well tolerated. Significant amelioration of the disease and damage was found with the use of SOD without any toxic effects.

• **SOD reduces inflammatory damage in joint tissue.** In a study published in *Acta Scandinavia,* several models of inflammation induced in laboratory animals were markedly inhibited by administration of SOD. In all cases, histological examination of the potential lesions revealed that treatment with SOD prevented accumulation of inflammatory cells.

Supplement Plan for Arthritis

Nutritional and herbal supplements differ from pharmaceutical drugs in that they can affect many systems simultaneously. These supplements are helpful in treating chronic illnesses such as arthritis because they contain a combination of ingredients that possess different beneficial actions. In fact, we have begun to test a new class of herbs and nutrients, phyto-anti-inflammatory drugs (PAIDs), for the treatment of chronic pain and degenerative conditions. Aspiring and other NSAIDs have been the cornerstones for treating inflammation and pain associated with arthritis, but have neglected the supportive role that dietary supplements provide—tissue support, antioxidant support, anti-inflammatory support! Many of these natural ingredients can serve as important adjuncts to traditional care or serve as a replacement for some drugs. We're learning that integrating supplements with conventional medicine is the best approach, since it gives us the benefits of both worlds, resulting in more effective, safer treatments. The following nutrients can be used as part of an integrated approach for arthritis:

Foundation Nutrient
SOD/gliadin, 200–500 I.U.

Joint and Tissue Support Nutrients
Chondroitin sulfate (Caldroitin™)
Glucosamine sulfate
S-adenosyl-methionine
N-acetyl-cysteine
Niacinamide

Anti-inflammatory Support Nutrients
Standardized stinging nettle extract
Standardized curcumin extract
Standardized perilla seed extract
Standardized boswellia extract
Standardized willow bark extract
Standardized devil's claw
Taxifolin
Resveratrol
Ursolic acid
Caffeic acid phenylester (CAPE)
Polyphenols (fruit, grape seed, pine bark)

Antioxidant Support
Full multiple antioxidant formula, with emphasis on both water-soluble antioxidants (such as vitamin C, polyphenols) and fat-soluble antioxidants (such as coenzyme Q_{10}, lipoic acid, vitamin E)

CHAPTER 2

SOD and Asthma

We can go for weeks without food, for days without water, but we can't go for more than a few minutes without breathing. Even so, we usually take breathing for granted. For most of us, air flows effortlessly in and out of our lungs, and we pay little attention. Not so for people with asthma, for whom the simple act of breathing can become an extraordinary effort. Nor is the condition a mere annoyance: Asthma can be devastating, even fatal. Almost 15 million Americans, including roughly 5 million children and young adults under the age of 18, suffer from asthma. Even more disturbing: Over the past 20 years, the incidence of childhood asthma has increased by more than 160%. Approximately 2 million hospital visits,

500,000 hospitalizations, and 5,000 deaths are directly related to asthma every year.

Take a Deep Breath

Asthma is a sometimes debilitating and painful condition marked by difficult breathing, caused by a narrowing or constricting of the bronchial passages in the lungs, which blocks air flow into the lungs. No one really knows what causes asthma, but it can be aggravated by a variety of stimuli, including allergens such as pollen, molds, foods, and pet hair; irritants such as smoke from tobacco or fires and chemicals such as household cleaners, paints,

---

Common Asthma Triggers

- Cold air
- Dust
- Strong fumes
- Exercise

- Inhaled irritants
- Emotional upset
- Smoke

Common Asthma Inducers

- Pollen (grass, tree, and weed)
- Molds

- Animal secretions (cat and horse tend to be the worst)
- House dust mites

---

and gasoline; infections in the respiratory system from colds or flus; certain medications such as non-steroidal anti-inflammatory drugs (NSAIDs); over-exertion, including exercise; emotional stress; and extreme air conditions such as dryness or cold. Asthma can be mild, occurring only during vigorous exercise, to severe, causing daily symptoms and requiring life restrictions.

People with asthma have hypersensitive airways that are almost always tender and at least slightly inflamed. When exposed to one of the above stimuli or triggers, they can suffer an asthma attack. An asthma attack is characterized by further narrowing of the airways, either through inflammation or bronchial constriction. In inflammation, the tissues swell in response to the allergen or other stimuli. In bronchial constriction, the muscles around the airways in the lungs contract tightly or go into spasm. Since people with asthma generally have hyper-responsive lung tissue—that is, their lungs over-react to stimuli. The resulting narrowing of the airways from either of these reactions makes breathing extremely difficult. Additionally, mucus buildup impedes the flow of oxygen and further exacerbates breathing difficulty.

Several conventional remedies including anti-inflammatories such as cortisone, and bronchial dilators, are used to treat asthma. Anti-inflamatories work by reducing the swelling in the tissue. Bronchial dilators work by relaxing the muscles, releasing their tightening grip on the airways and allowing the breath to pass easier again. Both types of drugs are effective, even necessary, for severe cases of asthma. However, they can cause a range of unpleasant side effects, including trembling, nervousness, increased heart rate, diarrhea, heartburn, loss of appetite, headaches, and upset stomach. Even worse, the long-term effects may include liver and kidney damage.

Radical News: The Role of Reactive Oxygen Species in Asthma

Although the exact causes of asthma aren't known, research has suggested that certain ROS free radicals, including superoxide, can damage lung tissue and lead to asthmatic conditions. Additionally, ROS exacerbate the symptoms of asthma, and the cumulative tissue damage caused by ROS free radicals can lead to progressively worse asthma. Studies have shown that when the epithelial cells, or the cells on the surface of the lining of the lungs and bronchia, become inflamed because of irritants such as cigarette smoke or illness, they tend to step up production of ROS free radicals. The overproduction of ROS free radicals is connected to some of the more dramatic symptoms of asthma, such as bronchial constriction and airway inflammation.

Here's how it works: When allergens, pathogens,

or other invaders attack tissues, the body stimulates the process of inflammation as a defensive mechanism. One of the signs of inflammation is swelling. When body tissue swells, it generates heat and sends out a signal to the immune system that something is wrong. The body responds in part by stepping up production of certain ROS free radicals, including superoxide, in an effort to kill off dangerous microorganisms that may have penetrated the defenses of the cell. And while ROS free radicals can destroy invaders, they can also lead to extensive tissue damage if left unchecked.

In people without asthma, the body slows its production of ROS once the invaders are in check, and all returns to normal. But in people with asthma, the production of ROS may not return to normal or safe levels. Normally, the body produces enough SOD and other antioxidants to reduce the levels of superoxide once the inflammatory situation is under control. But in the lungs of people with asthma, it works differently. People with asthma seem to be lacking the right mix of cellular defenses and protective antioxidants such as SOD. Until recently, the only way to stop an asthma attack was with drugs, which, as we've seen, have some pretty undesirable side effects. Now, however, studies are finding that SOD can offer effective protection against asthma attacks—with no side effects.

What the Studies Show

Studies have found that the body's levels of SOD and other antioxidants drop sharply immediately after the onset of an asthma attack. These findings suggest two things: First, the latent condition of asthma, like oversensitive tissues and allergies, predisposes the lungs to a deficiency of SOD in general and during an attack in particular. Because of this, superoxide becomes excessively abundant, goes beyond killing microorganisms, and starts to damage cells. This can become a vicious cycle, increasing the inflammation and worsening the attack. Additionally, studies have shown that significantly reduced levels of glutathione peroxidase (GSH-Px) are found in adults and children with asthma. GSH-Px is another important defense enzyme that is upregulated by the administration of SOD. Second, findings suggest that increasing the levels of SOD in the lungs can help prevent or treat asthma attacks and the symptoms of asthma—with less risk and at a lower cost than with drugs. While injectable bovine sources of SOD have been used in most studies, we now have the first vegetarian, orally absorbable form of this critically important enzyme—SOD/gliadin.

- **SOD helps fight respiratory disorders.** One study reported in the *American Journal of Physiology* set out to determine the usefulness of SOD in combating respiratory deficiency. Specifically, the researchers referred to difficulties in breathing in premature babies. Because of their underdeveloped lungs, these babies are at risk of developing chronic lung diseases such as bronchopulmonary dysplasia (BPD). The generally applied treatment for premature infants is oxygen supplementation. However, according to this study, even though the babies need oxygen to breathe, the increased levels of oxygen can lead to increased levels of oxygen free radicals, such as superoxide. The study suggests that supplemental SOD can fight superoxide-related tissue damage, ultimately preventing chronic lung diseases and other respiratory deficiency–related illnesses such as asthma.

• **SOD can relieve asthma symptoms.** Studies have generally found that signs of oxidative stress—including the production of ROS free radicals and their detrimental effects—are higher in people with asthma than without. In one study, reported in the *American Journal of Respiratory and Critical Care*, 44 patients varying from healthy to severely asthmatic were examined to determine their degree of oxidative stress. Researchers measured the amount of a certain substance that indicates high levels of oxidative stress and found that the worse the asthma, the higher the marker of oxidative stress. This suggests that higher free radical activity is associated with severe asthma and, further, that antioxidants such as SOD can help alleviate some of the symptoms of asthma. Another study, reported in *Vojnosanit Pregl*, examined 92 patients with asthma and 45 healthy subjects. The study found that people with more severe asthma had less defenses against free radicals than healthy people. Additionally, they found that patients taking antioxidants fared better than the patients not taking antioxidants— another indication that SOD can help fight asthma.

• **SOD is lost faster by people with asthma.** This study, reported in *The Lancet*, was based on the idea that ROS free radicals contribute to damage in the air passages, thus worsening the asthmatic response in people with asthma, and that damage from ROS free radicals is directly related to the level of antioxidants available in the lungs. In this study, an asthma attack was stimulated with an allergen—either grass or ragweed. The researchers found that immediately following the asthma attack, the levels of SOD in the asthma patient were significantly lower that in the control subjects. Additionally, 4 of the patients showed a continuous decrease in SOD levels for up to 48 hours after the attack. The strong relationship between the lower levels of SOD and asthma-symptom activity in these patients suggests that SOD could be a first-line defense against asthma attacks and that, by restoring SOD levels, it could protect the lung tissue from further oxidative damage.

• **The lung cells of people with asthma produce more ROS free radicals.** This study, reported in *Free Radical Biology and Medicine,* found that the lung cells of asthma patients produce more ROS than normal people. Additionally, blood tests done on asthma patients show lower-than-normal levels of SOD. The goal of the study was to show that SOD levels could be strong indicators of the inflammation that characterizes asthma. After studying 21 asthma patients and 17 controls, researchers found that not only were SOD levels lower in the asthma patients, but the increase of ROS in their lungs contributed to the increased levels of damage in the lining of the lungs. This effect is thought to increase the severity of asthma over time. The study suggests that SOD can reduce not only the symptoms of asthma, but also the progression of the condition itself.

• **SOD reduces the effects of allergens and chemicals.** Allergens and chemicals can trigger severe bronchial constriction, making breathing very difficult. Part of this process is a massive production of ROS as a reaction to these allergens. This production of ROS quickly becomes destructive and worsens the asthmatic response in a damaging cycle. One study, reported in the

American Journal of Respiratory and Critical Care Medicine, found that SOD could reduce the severity of an asthma attack triggered by allergens and chemicals. Researchers found that adequate levels of SOD reduced the constricting effect of the allergens and made breathing easier. These findings suggest that SOD can offer effective symptomatic treatment for asthma.

• **SOD levels are lower in asthma patients.** This study, reported in the *Journal of Asthma,* examined 25 people and found that asthma patients had lower levels of SOD than healthy patients. Researchers stated that although the exact relationship between antioxidants and asthma is still unclear, their clinical findings suggest that lower levels of antioxidants may contribute to the pathology of asthma—in other words, the physical symptoms that characterize asthma. This further implies that lower levels of SOD may actually contribute to causing asthma. Further, excess levels of ROS may stimulate and worsen inflammation in asthma patients, thus creating a damaging cycle. The study suggests that supplementing with SOD may stem the development of asthma.

• **SOD can protect the lungs from damage in allergic reactions.** Allergies are known to be a primary trigger of asthma attacks. A study reported in the *American Journal of Respiratory and Critical Care Medicine* found that when an allergic response occurs, cells in the lining of the lungs become inflamed, which triggers an increase in ROS production. According to the researchers, this additional production of ROS can contribute to lung tissue injury, as well as permanent changes in the airways, which may lead to diseases such as asthma. SOD can protect the lungs from that damage and reduce the occurrence of asthma and other airway-inflammatory diseases.

• **SOD can counter excess superoxide in asthma patients.** This study, reported in the *American Review of Respiratory Diseases,* examined the activity and concentration of monocytes, or inflammatory cells that occur in response to a trigger, in 18 asthma patients and 18 healthy controls. The monocytes in the asthma patients were found to release more superoxide than those in the control subjects, thus increasing the likelihood of tissue damage. Additionally, the asthma group had lower levels of SOD activity in response to the increase in superoxide. This suggests that superoxide activity unchecked by antioxidants plays a major role in the creation of asthma symptoms and the progression of the condition itself. Thus, SOD supplementation may help to relieve the symptoms of asthma and prevent further lung damage.

• **Superoxide derivatives cause inflammation in the lungs.** In the presence of antioxidants, superoxide creates several derivatives. Two of these are hydrogen peroxide and hydroxyl, both of which are types of ROS free radicals. Consequently, high concentrations of superoxide can lead to high concentrations of other damaging free radicals. A study reported in *Agent Actions* found more evidence to support the idea that these ROS free radicals create inflammation in the lungs that's related to asthma. In this study, researchers examined the effects of hydrogen peroxide and hydroxyl. Based on the premise that bronchial constriction is a primary symptom of an asthma attack, they set out to find the relationship of these ROS free radicals to airway constriction. What they found is that, like superoxide, these ROS free radicals contribute to a significant level of tissue inflammation in the airway, which leads to difficult breathing in people with asthma. SOD can counteract not only superoxide but also its derivatives, thus preventing inflammation and bronchial constriction.

Supplement Plan for Asthma

The use of dietary supplements for the prevention and treatment of asthma was limited until the use of SOD demonstrated positive results. Because asthma, like all other diseases, is a complex disease with many systems and pathways involved, the traditional single-magic-bullet approach will not be effective. SOD/gliadin along with other important natural antihistamines, anti-inflammatories, and supportive nutrients is the best approach to long-term, successful treatment. The following nutrients can be used as part of a treatment plan for asthma:

Foundation Nutrient
SOD/gliadin, 200–500 I.U.

Anti-inflammatory, Bronchodilator, and Antioxidant Support Nutrients
Glutamic acid
Quercetin
Troxerutin
Polyphenol extract (fruit, grape seed, pine bark)
Magnesium aspartate
Standardized ma huang extract
Standardized ginkgo biloba extract
Standardized licorice extract
Complete multiple antioxidant formula with special emphasis on vitamin A, vitamin E, and vitamin C
Complete vitamin B complex with special emphasis on nicotinamide, vitamin B_6, and vitamin B_{12}

CHAPTER 3

SOD AND CANCER

The most mysterious—and dreaded—of all illnesses, cancer has earned its reputation as a devastating, unstoppable disease. Nearly half a million people are expected to die from cancer this year. With approximately 1.2 million new cases annually, cancer is responsible for one out of four deaths—making it number two only to heart disease. And research has suggested that all of the cancer deaths every year, more than a third are the result of poor nutrition. The national cost of cancer is high: more than $107 billion a year, according to the National Institutes of Health (NIH). The good news is that SOD/gliadin is a new, natural substance that promotes internal defenses that may prevent or slow the development of cancer.

Anatomy of a Cancer Cell

Cancer is actually the name for a host of individual diseases that affect different parts of the body, each of which is characterized by the irregular and uncontrolled growth of *malignant* cells. "Malignant" simply describes a growth that invades and destroys the tissue in which is originated. Malignant cells are so devastating because they have the ability to *metastasize*, or spread to other parts of the body, unlike benign growths, which may interfere with the body's functioning because of the space they take up but aren't likely to destroy the tissue surrounding them or spread to other parts of the body.

Malignant cell production in the body can be caused by a variety of things, such as genetics, environmental toxins, and lifestyle factors, which can lead to a profusion of free radicals in the body. Ultimately, the result is damaged or mutated genes, which can lead to rapid, irregular, and uncontrolled cell growth—the condition we call cancer. Let's take a closer look.

One of the primary causes of cancer is genetics. That doesn't mean that if one of your parents had cancer, you're doomed, though you're probably at a higher risk than someone without a family history of cancer. When we say that the cause of a cancer is genetics, we mean that the malignancy originated because of a gene. Once a gene, which is normally responsible for producing healthy cells, becomes mutated and begins to produce unhealthy cells, it's called an *oncogene*. That damaged gene then stimulates the rapid and uncontrolled growth of malignant cancer cells.

Another class of genes called *tumor suppressor genes* is dedicated to preventing malignant growths in the body. The job of these genes is to stop cells with abnormal DNA structures from reproducing. But if the tumor suppressor genes are damaged by free radicals, they maybe unable to stop irregular cellular growth, which can then pervade the now defenseless body.

Another cause of cancer is radiation, including ultraviolet (UV) radiation from the sun. Prolonged, regular, and unprotected exposure to the sun can lead to skin cancer. UV rays, like sunlight, can cause what's called photooxidative damage, mutating or altering the DNA in skin cells, which can then lead to skin cancer.

Finally, of all the causes of cancer, lifestyle has probably the greatest impact on the propensity for cancer in an individual. The use of alcohol and tobacco, lack of antioxidant defense, poor dietary and exercise habits, and exposure to environmental toxins are all factors in the development of cancer.

Nearly 80% of all diagnosed cancers occur in people over the age of 55 for a simple reason: The longer your body has been around, the more toxins it has accumulated and the more the cells have been damaged. And as the body ages, its ability to repair damage is lessened. Unfortunately, your chances of getting cancer are pretty good. Over the course of a lifetime, men have about a 50% chance of getting some form of cancer and women have about a 33% chance.

If you do get cancer, you can expect your doctor to recommend some or all of the three conventional treatments, none of which has much appeal. *Surgery* involves removing the malignant tumor or cancerous tissue, as well as a "buffer" of healthy tissue around it to ensure that all the cancerous growth is removed. This can be an effective treatment for contained cancers that haven't metastasized. *Chemotherapy* is the process of using powerful drugs that target and destroy rapidly dividing cells. The hope is that the drug will eliminate the cancer without causing irreparable damage to the body's healthy cells. Unfortunately, some healthy cells in the body, such as those of the liver, kidney, and hair, are rapidly dividing. That's why chemotherapy patients often lose their hair. *Radiation therapy* works by mutating the malignant cells so they can no longer rapidly divide. Ironically, this therapy uses the same process that may have created the cancer-causing mutations in the first place.

How Free Radicals Cause Cancer

What causes cancer? No one knows the exact mechanisms, but free radicals have been strongly implicated in the cause and progression of this disease. ROS free radicals and superoxide free radicals, in particular, have been associated with nearly every kind of cancer studied.

Earlier, we discussed free radicals and the kinds of cellular devastation to which they can lead. As we've seen, an imbalance of free radicals can result from several causes, including diet, lifestyles, and environmental toxins. Usually, the body produces enough antioxidants, such as SOD, to balance out the overproduction of free radicals. But when the ratio of antioxidants to free radicals is lowered, damage quickly begins to occur. Once an overload of ROS free radicals exists, the cellular devastation that leads to cancer can occur.

As we've seen, ROS free radicals can alter a cell's DNA by robbing it of electrons, resulting in a mutated genetic code within the cell. Because DNA is the template for cell reproduction, when a cell with mutated DNA replicates, it will produce other mutated cells. The unhappy result is rapid cell division and uncontrollable growth, or what we call malignant cancer.

ROS free radicals can also damage a cell's membrane. The cell membrane acts like a barrier, the same as our skin, to protect the interior of the cell, including its DNA, from free radicals and other harmful substances. If the walls are damaged, the exchange of nutrients and waste products is impaired and the cell becomes toxic. In addition, the cellular walls contain fats, or lipids. If ROS free radicals attack the walls of the cell, the lipids in the cell

How Cancer Happens

How does cancer happen? It's a complicated network of factors and events, but here's the simple version. Cancer generally begins with an external or internal stimulus that promotes the production of free radicals. Among the most dangerous and damaging kinds of free radicals are ROS free radicals, such as superoxide. These insidious free radicals can cause a slew of cellular damage and, ultimately, genetic damage within the cells.

As we've seen, once the genes of a cell are damaged, the directions for cell reproduction are destroyed and the gene begins to produce new cells at a rapid and uncontrollable rate. The first manifestation of that growth is a lesion, or a small cluster of abnormal cells. The next stage is a tumor. When tumors release malignant cells into the bloodstream and other parts of the body, the cancer spreads.

walls can themselves become a type of ROS free radical called *lipid peroxyl radicals (LPRs)*. These LPRs continue to perpetrate cellular damage in a vicious cycle. The cell's DNA is then susceptible to free radical damage and may become mutated.

Lipids are essential in the process of cellular communication, which takes place on the membranes of the cells. Cells communicate by the exchange of chemical signals across the cell membranes, and some of those communications tell the cells when to reproduce. If the communication goes amok, cells begin to reproduce incorrectly. The cell walls also contain enzymes, protein structures that influence a number of biological reactions, including cellular communication and growth. If those enzymes are damaged by ROS free radicals, they can send improper signals and may contribute to uncontrollable growth—or cancer—in damaged cells.

ROS free radicals are also believed to inhibit normal cell *apoptosis,* or death. Normally, when a cell becomes damaged from free radicals or toxicity, the body sends out certain chemicals that order cellular suicide, to prevent these dangerous cellular mutations from spreading. ROS free radicals can interfere with the body's ability to order a cell's death.

Finally, ROS free radicals also promote the motility, or movement, of cancer cells. If cancer cells are moving through the body, they're more likely to reproduce in other areas. The state of dispersement of cancer cells throughout the body is usually the final stage in the progression of cancer. And if the cancer has been resistant to treatments such as chemotherapy, there is usually little left that can be done to protect the body from continued devastation.

To summarize, damaging free radicals are a result of diet, lifestyle, inadequate antioxidant defense, environmental toxins, and normal body processes, and they're usually kept in check by antioxidants. If there aren't enough antioxidants in the body, the free radicals can proliferate and cause immense damage to the cells. Luckily, studies have shown that SOD can help prevent the development of cancer and can slow its spread once it has developed. Additionally, SOD can offset many of the negative effects of conventional cancer treatments and make those treatments more effective.

What the Studies Show

Because of the devastating effects of cancer, researchers are tirelessly searching for clues to how to prevent and, ultimately, cure cancer. What they're finding is that because ROS free radicals are so strongly associated with cancer, SOD can inhibit metastasis, slow tumor growth, and prevent the initial cellular damage that can lead to cancer in the first place. Additionally, SOD can help protect and repair healthy tissue that's damaged by chemotherapy and radiation treatments.

- **SOD slows the spread of cancer.** In order for a tumor to metastasize, malignant cells must detach from the tumor, invade surrounding tissue, dodge the defenses of the immune system, and infiltrate the bloodstream. Sounds like a challenge. But when these cells are dividing at uncontrollable rates and the body's defenses are lowered, metastasis can happen very quickly. In an in vitro (test tube) study of human cancer cells, researchers found that SOD significantly reduced metastasis. The hope is that in the human body, SOD can help prevent the spread of existing cancers.

• **SOD makes chemotherapy more effective.** Adriamycin is a strong drug used in conventional chemotherapy treatments. The same study mentioned above found that not only did SOD inhibit the spread of tumors, but when it was combined with adriamycin, the results were even better. If SOD enhances the effectiveness of adriamycin, it's possible that, ultimately, less harsh chemotherapy drugs need to be used. Additionally, researchers suggest that by adjusting adriamycin levels in a "cocktail" with SOD, the exact level of tumor-inhibiting therapy can be achieved.

• **SOD inhibits growth of breast cancer.** Once cells become cancerous, one goal is to prevent them from growing. In this in vitro study, researchers found that SOD helped to suppress tumor growth of human breast cancer. Apparently, SOD reduces the effectiveness of certain chemical substances that are responsible for the reproduction of damaged genes leading to malignant cells. Because damaged cells in cancer-

ous tumors can't reproduce effectively when
SOD is present, cancerous growths can be inhibited.

• **SOD may prevent skin cancer.** Another study
tested the effectiveness of SOD treatment in
combination with exposure to UV radiation. As
we've seen, UV rays, such as sunlight, can damage the skin and possibly result in skin cancer.
Furthermore, even a one-time exposure to UV
radiation can cause a significant decrease in the
antioxidant SOD for up to 72 hours after exposure. In this study, the researchers divided the
study participants into two groups. They found
that the untreated group showed a significant decline in SOD levels. By comparison, the test
group that was pretreated with SOD had an increase of SOD activity initially and maintained a
higher level of SOD production for nearly 72
hours. The study implies that SOD not only can
prevent skin cancer, as well as other skin diseases,
it can actually increase the body's ability to manufacture SOD.

• **SOD prevents tissue damage in radiation therapy.** The treatment of bladder cancer with radiation often results in other damaging conditions,
such as cystitis, a painful inflammation of the
bladder that can be accompanied by the passing
of blood. The incredibly destructive force of radiation therapy can also lead to subcutaneous, or

inner tissue, damage to noncancerous areas. SOD can help prevent damage from radiation. In a study of 448 bladder cancer patients undergoing radiation therapy, researchers found that the patients treated with SOD had a much lower incidence of cystitis. In addition, further tests showed that the SOD group had significantly less cellular damage in the deeper layers of the skin. The study suggests that SOD used in conjunction with radiation therapy not only can prevent immediate damage from the radiation, but can also protect against damage that may occur later.

• **SOD can protect against and reverse fibrosis.** Radiation therapy can also cause fibrosis, a painful thickening and scarring of the connective tissue that can impair mobility. Radiation-induced fibrosis (RIF) occurs more frequently when the skin is double-dosed with radiation, as when treatment areas overlap or second treatments are given for recurrent tumors. In a study of cancer patients being treated with radiation, researchers found that SOD helped relieve RIF. Patients were injected with SOD at the site of the fibrosis over a specified period of time during the course of their treatment and were then followed for an average of 5 years. All of them showed improvement in the condition of their fibrotic tissues, often in the form of softening and relaxing of the tissue. Additionally, in cases where the fibrotic connective tissue was impairing movement because of its proximity to bones and joints, free movement was restored.

• **SOD prevents skin damage in the treatment of lung cancer.** Other anti-cancer therapies can damage healthy tissues as well. Bleomycin (BLM), a drug that's used in the chemotherapy treatment of lung cancer, Hodgkin's disease, and certain other cancers, is known for causing fibrosis. This study found that SOD, when used in conjunction with BLM, can protect tissues from fibrosis, without interfering with the action of the BLM.

• **Low levels of SOD point to more aggressive tumors.** Certain cancer-causing agents such as nickel and lead—usually found in cigarette smoke and air pollution—are devastating toxins that can deplete SOD levels in the body. Because they are very difficult to eliminate, their residue is often found in cancerous lung tissue. A study of 38 lung cancer patients found that lower levels of SOD were associated with higher levels of these toxic metals, as well as more aggressive tumors in the lungs. If can be presumed that if higher levels of SOD were present, the deleterious actions of these toxins and tumors might be lessened.

• **SOD works with other anti-tumor factors.** OK432 is a powerful anti-tumor compound used in conventional cancer treatments. In a study published in the *International Journal of Cancer,* researchers found that when white blood cells were treated with OK432, the body's own production of a certain kind of SOD tended to increase. This study supports the theory that SOD is one of the important preliminary defenses against the invasion and spread of cancer in the white blood cells and that it enhances the actions of other anti-cancer drugs.

• **SOD may protect against gastric cancer.** Gastric cancer is one of the most painful and devastating kinds of cancer. A clinical study with 81 participants looked at the role of SOD in people with gastric cancer. Blood samples from patients with gastritis and atypical hyperplasia, two conditions that often are early indicators of gastric cancer, showed lowered levels of SOD. Additionally, the group with gastric cancer showed significantly reduced levels of SOD. The researchers propose that SOD may play an important role in protecting against gastric cancer and the free radical superoxide by preventing abnormal cells from actually becoming cancerous. Additionally, the researchers postulate that low levels of SOD may be an early indicator of a cancerous condition.

• **Cancer patients have lower levels of SOD.** Other researchers had similar findings after testing patients with gastric, colorectal, hepatic, or pancreatic cancer. The researchers found lower levels of SOD in these cancer patients as compared to healthy volunteers. Previous studies had found that blood levels of SOD are reduced by carcinogens and the toxic effects of the free radical superoxide. This study further suggests a direct relationship between the levels of SOD and the incidence of cancer.

Supplement Plan for Cancer

The use of dietary supplements for the prevention and treatment of cancer is gaining widespread acceptance as an adjunct to traditional treatments. Because cancer, like all other diseases, is a complex illness with many systems and pathways involved, the traditional single-magic-bullet approach often is not effective and in the best interests of the patient. The following nutrients can be used as part of an integrated treatment approach for cancer:

Foundation Nutrient
  SOD/gliadin, 200–500 I.U.

Nutrients to Prevent Muscle/Tissue Loss
  Undenatured Whey Protein
  OKG (ornithine alpha ketoglutarate)
  Branched Chain Amino Acids
  Nucleotides
  L-Glutamine

Antioxidant Support
  Beta Glucans
  Polyphenols
  Coenzyme Q10
  Nucleotides
  High Immunoglobulin Whey Protein
  L-lysine
  L-Glutamine
  Full multiple antioxidant formula, with empha-
    sis on both water soluble and fat soluble anti-
    oxidants

  Immunomodulating/Antimicrobial Herbs:
    olive leaf, elderberry, scutellaria, andro-
    graphis, oregano, basil, reishi/shiitake &
    maitake mushrooms, tumeric, astragalus, cat's
    claw, isoflavones, modified citrus pectin

Mitochondrial/Energy Support
  Coenzyme Q10
  D-Ribose
  L-Carnitine
  MCT (medium chain triglycerides)
  L-Glutamine

CHAPTER 4

SOD AND CARDIOVASCULAR SUPPORT

The heart is possibly the most important organ in the body. It is physiologically responsible for our lives, and we have conferred upon it great psychological and emotional meaning as well. We call those we love "sweetheart" or "heartthrob." Our "hearts race" when we are excited. And when love is lost, we are "heartbroken." As romantic and impulsive as our tender phrases make the heart sound, the organ itself is a practical and steadfast servant, pumping endlessly and tirelessly day after day, year after year. Or, at least, until problems break its steady rhythm.

A Heartbreaking Story

In spite of newspaper headlines about cancer
and acquired immune deficiency syndrome (AIDS),
it's heart disease that's the real killer. More than
one million Americans a year suffer heart attacks.
Break that number down and you'll find it trans-
lates into about one heart attack every 20 seconds—
a third of which lead to death. The good news is
that scientific advancements have shed new light on
the prevention and treatment of heart disease, with
radical new, *natural* therapies that center around
preventing inflammation and the use of antioxidants. One in particular—SOD—has been shown
to protect the heart from damage and disease. We'll
talk more about that later. First, let's take a closer
look at this vital organ.

The heart has a monumental job: to supply the
entire body with oxygen-rich blood, necessary for
the survival of every cell. The heart itself is a mus-
cular pump about the size of a fist, located in the
chest just left of center behind the sternum. It
works by collecting oxygen-depleted blood from
the body and pumping it to the lungs, where the
blood can drop off carbon dioxide and pick up
fresh oxygen. That oxygen-rich blood is then col-
lected again by the heart and carried throughout
the body to nourish the cells via a complex network
of arteries. The arteries serve as superhighways for
the blood and as such are absolutely vital to cardiovascular health.

The Heart of the Matter: The Vital Role of the Arteries

Though the heart beats without much external impetus from us, it shouldn't be neglected. Most important for a healthy heart are healthy arteries. The *coronary arteries* in particular need to be clear and strong, since they're the conduit of the blood, oxygen, and nutrients that nourish the heart muscle itself. The general condition of unhealthy arteries is called *atherosclerosis,* or hardening of the arteries. Atherosclerosis is the progressive buildup of materials on the interior lining of the arteries. It can start as early as childhood and typically accelerates dramatically during the 30s and 40s, with no obvious symptoms. By the time we're in our mid-50s, our arteries may be hopelessly blocked. The possible result is fatal illness, including heart attack and stroke.

You may think you know what causes atherosclerosis—bacon cheeseburgers with extra mayo, right? Not necessarily. In spite of all we've read, the precipitating factor behind atherosclerosis isn't just fat and cholesterol—it's *oxidized* fat and cholesterol, as well as high insulin levels and oxidized iron, minerals, and other compounds. That's how free radicals fit in. In short, at the heart of atherosclerosis is free radical damage to fat, cholesterol, and other compounds that starts the process of atherosclerosis. Also, remember that the heart is a muscle. Muscles require energy to work and anything that interferes with that production of energy can cause damage.

So, it *is* about fat and cholesterol, but it's not *only* about fat and cholesterol. Let's look at cardiovascular disease and the role of free radicals, oxidation, cholesterol, and general energy production in the body.

A Radical Change: The Role of Free Radicals in Heart Disease

As we discussed in earlier chapters, a free radical is a molecule with an unbalanced number of electrons to protons. In order to rebalance its charges, a newly created free radical steals an electron from another molecule. The result is a devastating chain reaction that ultimately damages cells and the tissues they make up. Without antioxidant protection, the continual assault that free radicals wage on the body can ultimately lead to disease, one of which is atherosclerosis.

In atherosclerosis, free radicals cause a rip or a tear in the arterial wall. In an attempt to repair itself, the arterial wall snatches cholesterol and other substances from passing blood to coat the damaged area. If the old wound is reopened by more free radicals, more cholesterol and other substances are piled on top, forming what's called *plaque*. Over time, a buildup of plaque begins to narrow the artery and make it less flexible. This narrowing and inflexibility can seriously affect the body's ability to receive blood and make it harder for the heart to pump blood through the body, thus creating a strain on the heart muscle.

Free radicals can also damage the DNA. Considered the "blueprints" of cells, these crucial molecules are responsible for providing instructions for the production of new, healthy cells. A cell reproduces by rapidly doubling its DNA and then splitting into two separate cells, each with a complete DNA molecule. When a free radical collides with a DNA molecule, it can mutate the DNA, causing the directions for cell reproduction to be lost or altered. If the directions are lost, the cell will die. If the directions are altered, the mutated cell can begin to reproduce as an unhealthy cell, including cancer, or another abnormal growth, such as a tumor in the wall of an artery, which can restrict blood flow and cut down on the heart's supply of oxygen.

Fat Chance: The Cholesterol Problem

So that's the free radical story. Now, how does cholesterol fit into the picture? Let's take a look at the fat we love to hate and how it contributes to heart disease.

Cholesterol is a fatlike substance that does have many important functions in the body, including the manufacture of many hormones. Because it's fat-soluble, cholesterol is unable to dissolve in the blood and move about, so it attaches to compounds known as *lipoproteins*, which are like little bags that float through the blood and carry cholesterol molecules around the body. There are several types of lipoprotein cholesterol compounds, including low-density lipoprotein (LDL) cholesterol and high-density lipoprotein (HDL) cholesterol. LDL cholesterol is low in density because it's puffed up with cholesterol. LDLs have a tendency to drop off cholesterol wherever they land, including in the arteries, hence the name "bad cholesterol." HDL cholesterol is high in density because it's compressed, like a bag with the air sucked out. When an HDL connects to a cell wall, it opens and expands, accepting excess cholesterol from the cell. It then hops back into the bloodstream and transports the cholesterol back to the liver, where it's processed and excreted, hence the term "good cholesterol."

Cholesterol can damage the heart in a couple of ways. As we saw earlier, if free radicals damage an arterial wall, cholesterol is deposited over the "wound" and, over time, can cause plaque buildup and narrowing of the artery. More insidious is the interplay between cholesterol and oxygen.

The Very Air We Breathe: The Role of Oxidation in Cardiovascular Disease

When we hear the word "oxygen," we think of fresh air and a source of life. But in an irony of nature, oxygen can turn against us and cause untold damage in the body, in a process known as *oxidation* and the formation of *oxygen free radicals*.

Earlier we saw that a molecule is made up of two or more atoms abound together, so an oxygen molecule (O_2) is made up of two oxygen atoms. Each oxygen atom is made up of eight protons and eight electrons. Again, through a variety of factors, including bad eating and lifestyle habits, an oxygen atom may lose or gain an electron. The oxygen atom that has lost an electron now contains eight protons and seven electrons, so it's disproportionately balanced to the positive.

Nature loves balance, and oxygen molecules are no exception. So the unbalanced, positively charged oxygen molecule craves an electron to replace the one that was lost. Like a missile, it seeks out and smashes into another atom, scooping up an electron to restore its own balance. The atom into which it crashed is now short an electron and itself becomes a free radical. This process can continue indefinitely, in the cascade effect we mentioned earlier, causing significant cellular damage.

There's another version of the story. An oxygen molecule can also *gain* an electron and become negatively charged. These molecules, called *superoxides*, are considered the most potentially damaging free radical. Because of its chemical structure, a superoxide requires three electrons to rebalance itself. When it snatches those three electrons from other molecules, it creates even more imbalance. Also, it tends to perpetuate itself rapidly, creating more superoxides, so it has the potential to do a lot of damage. Both these kinds of free radicals are termed *reactive oxygen species (ROS),* dangerous compounds that have been associated with all kinds of degenerative processes, including cardiovascular disease, Alzheimer's disease, Parkinson's disease, arthritis, and cancer.

Back to cholesterol for a moment. Cholesterol is bad enough as it is, but when it becomes oxidized, it's much more dangerous. The cholesterol compound contains oxygen, which can become a free radical in the process we've just seen. Cholesterol travels in high concentrations in the bloodstream, so if its oxygen molecules have become free radicals, it carries the potential for incredible damage.

Energetic Players: The Role of Mitochondria in Superoxide

As you read this book, your eyes move across the words and your fingers turn the pages—tiny movements we take for granted. But even the smallest motion requires a source of energy. Let's look at energy production in the body and how it's related to other factors that influence cardiovascular disease.

The cells in our body contain *mitochondria,* little engines that produce the energy that make cells and, ultimately, tissue and muscles work. Without these microscopic generators, we wouldn't be able to move our bodies. Mitochondria use absorbed nutrients and oxygen to create energy and water. In the process of producing energy, superoxide is created.

It's a very normal part of the body's process and usually doesn't cause any problems. But when there are toxins in the nutrients and oxygen the mitochondria are trying to process, superoxides can be generated in excessive amounts. And, in terms of cardiovascular health, mitochondria are highly concentrated in the heart, so if they're producing excessive amounts of superoxide, the potential for damage to the heart is tremendous. Additionally, when tissue in the heart muscle is cut off from blood and oxygen, which can happen when arteries are blocked, the concentration of free radicals in the mitochondria increases significantly.

It's a heartbreaking story, but there is a solution, in the form of compounds that fight free radicals, especially superoxide. They're called *antioxidants*. As the name implies, antioxidants are designed to counter the highly damaging oxidative process we talked about earlier. They work by restoring the electron balance in free radicals, while themselves converting into a neutral substance. There are dozens of antioxidants, each one responsible for rebalancing a specific free radical. Our focus is on one particular antioxidant, SOD.

The Super Role of SOD

The body is a shrewd mechanism, and it knows how to take care of itself. It realizes that superoxide is a natural by-product of energy production in the mitochondria, so it also knows how to produce SOD, and enzyme designed to eliminate superoxide, SOD can *dismutate*, or balance, two superoxide molecules in a clever little molecular dance. Let's look at how it works:

1. Superoxide molecules are created as a by-product of energy production in the mitochondria.
2. SOD bumps into two of those superoxide molecules, each of which has an extra electron.
3. SOD removes the extra electron from superoxide molecule A and gives that extra electron to superoxide molecule B. A is now rebalanced and does not pose a threat to the body.
4. Superoxide molecule B now has two electrons, so it attracts two protons, which are hydrogen atoms, to balance itself. The result is one oxygen molecule and one hydrogen peroxide molecule.
5. Finally, the hydrogen peroxide, a much milder compound, can be converted into oxygen and water by an enzyme called catalase, which is naturally produced by the body.

This process is happening all the time in our bodies, usually at a manageable level—assuming there's enough SOD in our bodies to keep the damage at bay. But if the body is weakened by a poor diet, stress, disease, environmental toxins, or unhealthy lifestyle habits such as smoking, inadequate rest, and lack of exercise, SOD levels can become depleted. And SOD levels naturally decline with age. The result? It's harder for the body to control the levels of damaging superoxides. The good news is that SOD/gliadin supplementation, in combination with a healthy lifestyle, can help avoid a cardiovascular crisis.

What the Studies Show

All this information is well and good. But what does the science say? Studies have shown that SOD has several beneficial actions on cardiovascular health: It can control cholesterol levels, regulate heart contractions, reduce the levels of free radicals in the heart, and protect the heart against damage. And unlike some of the drugs that are used to address high cholesterol and other cardiovascular issues, SOD is free of side effects and much less expensive. While most of the following studies had to rely on injecting bovine extracts of SOD, today we can successfully employ the first bioavailable, vegetarian form of this critically important enzyme—SOD/gliadin.

• **SOD regulates cholesterol and triglycerides.** SOD has been shown to have positive effects on cholesterol, especially in cases where cholesterol levels were raised by the dietary intake of fats and cholesterol. In the body, fats are stored as *triglycerides*. High levels of triglycerides, as well as of cholesterol, have been consistently associated with increased risk of heart disease. A French study showed that SOD can actually normalize both triglycerides and total cholesterol levels. In other words, the radio between HDL cholesterol and VLDL (very-low-density lipoprotein) cholesterol can reach optimal levels with SOD supplementation, thus reducing the risk of atherosclerosis.

• **SOD reduces free radicals in the heart.** When blocked coronary arteries cut off blood and oxygen from the heart, tissue is damaged. That damaged tissue is called *ischemic*. When blood suddenly returns to the heart, it can cause irregular contraction of the heart muscle, a dangerous condition called *fibrillation* that can result in heart attack and death. Both ischemia and fibrillation are associated with dramatically higher levels of free radicals. A study by Japanese researchers showed that SOD was able to significantly reduce the levels of free radicals in ischemic tissue and in cases of fibrillation. Additionally, SOD appears to have a calming and regulatory effect on the heart and has been associated with lower levels of fibrillation. And, as we saw earlier, SOD may help prevent or alleviate the initial condition of blockage.

• **SOD reduces tissue damage to the heart.** In surgical situations, such as transplants, free radicals are a formidable foe. In these crisis situations, they accelerate tissue and organ death, not just in the heart, but also in other vital areas, such as the lungs. As we saw earlier, the heart is a transfer station for exchanging oxygen-and-nutrient-rich blood with "dirty" blood. In a study conducted at Johns Hopkins University, researchers found that administering SOD in surgical and transplant situations greatly reduces tissue damage in the heart and other vital organs. The SOD probably increases the life span of these vital tissues by neutralizing free radicals that could inflict serious and permanent cellular damage.

Other studies have similarly shown that SOD can protect the heart from damage by stemming the accumulation of oxygen free radicals and allowing the heat to recover faster.

• **SOD protects against heart damage caused by anti-cancer drugs.** Certain pathologies, such as cancer, require the use of drugs that can damage the ability of the mitochondria to produce energy efficiently. Because mitochondria are the source of cellular energy, the result is damage to cells and, thus, damage to muscle tissue. This can result in a cardiovascular disease known as cardiomyopathy. The damaged muscle is classified as either *hypertrophic,* meaning it's thick and swollen; *dilated,* meaning it's thin and weak; or *restricted,* meaning its movement is impaired. One study of the potent anti-cancer drug adriamycin found that supplemental SOD prevented cardiomyopathy and would be a useful natural treatment for patients battling cancer.

In the case of dilated cardiomyopathy, the natural production of SOD is slowed or stopped, which creates a vicious cycle of destruction. Because free radicals cause cardiomyopathy in the first place, once the damage occurs and SOD production is slowed or halted, the damage is perpetuated. A study conducted at Emory University School of Medicine found that supplementing with SOD can help stem this damage, allowing the heart muscle to begin its natural process of repair.

• **SOD supplementation may allow the body's SOD to replicate itself.** In a study reported in *FASEB,* researchers found that SOD in atherosclerotic plaque had damaged DNA. As we've seen, when DNA is damaged, a cell is unable to reproduce itself effectively. Thus, SOD molecules that had been damaged by oxidation are unable to reproduce themselves, lowering overall SOD levels in the body. Again, it's a vicious cycle: When SOD is needed the most, as in the case of atherosclerosis, the levels are lowered. Supplemental SOD not only may protect the heart against free radicals, but may also prevent damage to the body's stores of SOD, allowing them to replicate and provide further protection against heart disease.

- **SOD helps regulate heart contractions.** The heart pumps in two phases. In the first phase, blood is pumped into the heart. In the second phase, blood is pumped from the heart into the lungs and throughout the body. Regular contractions are essential to nourish the heart, as well as the rest of the body, with oxygen-rich blood. Additionally, if contractions are irregular, the result can be a fibrillation, a potentially dangerous condition. A study by Chinese researchers found that supplementing with SOD helps smooth and regulate the contractions of the heart and increase its output of blood.

Supplement Plan for Cardiovascular Disease

The use of dietary supplements for the treatment of cardiovascular disorders is crucial to the success of patient rehabilitation. Since cardiovascular disease is diverse (hypertension, atherosclerosis, arrhythmias, etc.), it requires specific manipulation of several dietary ingredients, rather than a single-magic-bullet approach. The following nutrients can be used as part of an integrated treatment approach for cardiovascular care:

Foundation Nutrient
SOD/gliadin, 200–500 I.U.

Cardio Support Nutrients
L-carnitine
Taurine
Coenzyme Q_{10}
Lipoic acid
Polyphenols (fruit, grape seed, pine bark)
Hawthorne extract
Calcium and magnesium
Vitamin B_6, vitamin B_{12}, and folic acid

Cholesterol Lowering Support Nutrients
Soy isoflavones and saponins
Pantetheine
Fenugreek seed extract
Tocotrienols and tocopherols
Guggulipid
Oat bran
No-flush niacin
Red yeast

CHAPTER 5

SOD AND IMMUNITY

Modern life can be an extreme challenge, even on a good day. Our bodies are continually bombarded by pollution, pesticides, chlorinated water, radiation, plastics, hormones, antibiotics, fluoride, heavy metals, and more. The result? An overload on the immune system, which leaves us tired, stressed, and more prone to illnesses and disorders, from allergies and arthritis to AIDS. SOD/gliadin, the master cellular defense antioxidant enzyme, offers a safe and effective way to boost the body's natural defenses.

The Main Defense

Exposure to bugs and viruses is an everyday occurrence. As we breathe, eat, and move through the world, our bodies are exposed to countless pathogens on a daily basis. Our immune system is what protects us from the potential dangers of the external world. On the outermost level, it begins with the skin, a generally intact sheath that keeps foreign objects out of our bodies. And if external defenses are penetrated, internal defenses step in. For example, the digestive system helps eliminate any pathogens that may sneak in with food. At a microscopic level, the immune system is composed of an elaborate, highly trained team of special cells that work around the clock, if necessary, to defend the body.

Under normal circumstances, the immune system fights off harmful bacteria, viruses, and other pathogens with little problem. But if the immune system is damaged, certain illnesses that contribute to a profusion of free radicals such as ROS can wreak havoc. SOD/gliadin can strengthen the immune system, preventing it from being damaged by ROS free radicals and possibly helping protect it against the effects of illnesses and conditions that could devastate it, including human immunodeficiency virus (HIV) and acquired immune deficiency syndrome (AIDS).

According to the National Institutes of Health in Washington, D.C., almost 35 million people worldwide live with HIV or AIDS. HIV is a virus that attacks and reproduces in the immune system, destroying important immune cells like the T cells and leaving the body open to other infections. AIDS is the state in which the body has manifested fatal infection or disease as a result of a weakened immune system. Both diseases are reaching epidemic proportions in sub-Saharan Africa, where the incidence of infection is exceeding 10% of adults in some countries. In the United States, the Centers for Disease Control and Prevention estimates the number of current cases at 650,000 to 900,000, with 200,000 as yet undiagnosed.

HIV and AIDS are so devastating because they directly attack the immune system. In most viral illnesses, the virus attacks a part of the body, such as the red blood cells or the muscle cells, and the immune system cells come to the rescue. In the case of HIV, the virus attacks the immune system itself, leaving the body completely defenseless. If HIV progresses into AIDS, the probability of death is high, but not from the AIDS itself. Rather, AIDS patients usually die from infections such as pneumonia that the exhausted immune system can no longer fight off.

The Battlefield in the Body

The body is equipped with a vast array of defense mechanisms that protect against harmful external factors, including bacteria, viruses, and environmental toxins. The immune system works in two primary ways: It disables foreign invaders and it repairs damaged tissue and cells. If the body's system becomes overloaded by external factors, including poor diet, cigarette smoking, or exposure to toxic chemicals, the immune system is unable to keep up. And when defenses are down, the body is more prone to harmful external influences.

The immune response is an extraordinarily complex process that's beyond the scope of this book, so let's just look at the basics. A healthy immune system depends in large part on functioning and abundant *T cells*. *Helper T cells* facilitate communication and stimulate an immune attack. If the attack isn't called off at some point, the immune cells may turn on the body instead, as in autoimmune disorders such as lupus and rheumatoid arthritis. *Suppressor T cells* send the signals to halt the attack once an invader is dead, thus preventing the body from being damaged.

Macrophages are cells that capture and "digest" foreign invaders. Moving through the body like a Pac Man, the macrophages gobble up invaders and present them to the helper T cells. The T cells then initiate one of many complex reactions. Most commonly, T cells send a signal to *B cells,* which produce antibodies that kill foreign invaders. Once the danger is over, suppressor T cells call for a cease-fire.

It appears that HIV damages the body by killing T cells, thus impairing communication. Further, there are different degrees of infection with HIV.

Whatever the course of treatment, the goal is to minimize the level of destruction in the body from HIV. Here's where SOD comes in. Some research has found that oxidative stress exacerbates the action of HIV in the body and that the same ROS free radicals that contribute to cancer, heart disease, asthma, allergies, neurological damage, and other disorders also play a role in increasing the expression of HIV. Again, in the case of oxidative stress, the balance of oxidants to antioxidants is unfavorable and leads to excessive cellular damage. And in the case of HIV, it's a double-edged sword. HIV contributes to oxidative stress, which in turn can exacerbate the HIV condition. Not only is this relationship damaging in itself, but it also provides the opportunity for subsequent infections and other ROS-related illnesses.

One major way ROS contribute to the proliferation of HIV is by killing immune cells, a process called *apoptosis,* or cell death. Apoptosis is a natural process that happens constantly in the body—as old or damaged cells die, new cells are produced. The immune system helps with apoptosis by ridding the body of damaged cells before they can mutate and become cancerous. But ROS can prematurely damage cells. If immune cells become prematurely damaged by ROS and killed off by apoptosis at high rates, the body can become defenseless.

Apoptosis of T cells is characteristic of HIV and AIDS, and ROS, like superoxide, contributes to this event. Many studies have investigated possible ways to prevent this anti-immune conspiracy between ROS and HIV. Without fail, most of the research has suggested that antioxidants such as SOD can be beneficial. By fighting the damaging effects of ROS on the cells, SOD can limit, and even stabilize or reduce, the expression of HIV. Nobody is saying that SOD can prevent or cure AIDS, but it might help, as an auxiliary treatment, to quell the fury of cellular devastation. Further, if SOD can support the immune system against a foe such as HIV, it can likely help with other immune-related difficulties and illnesses.

What the Studies Show

Much of the research available of SOD and the immune system centers around HIV and antioxidants. Because the immune system has a more general function in the body, protecting us from disease and keeping us healthy in a myriad of ways, the clearest observations of the relationship among ROS, SOD, and the immune system are found in studying HIV and AIDS. But research also makes associations between oxidative stress and the overall strength of the immune system. In general, studies suggest that SOD can offset the damage done by ROS, preventing damage to the immune system, and consequently help delay or prevent the onset of degenerative diseases and immune-related conditions such as HIV and AIDS.

- **SOD levels are lowered in patients with pneumonia.** A study reported in *Clinical Chemistry* found that superoxide levels were higher and SOD levels were lower in patients with pneumonia. The study included 91 people of varied ages and sex, and consisted of compromised groups (lung cancer) and noncompromised groups with and without pneumonia. Compared to the healthy controls, the compromised groups showed lower levels of SOD and higher levels of superoxide. The compromised groups with pneumonia showed even less SOD and more superoxide. The study shows a relationship between immune-stressing illness and levels of SOD. And because higher levels of superoxide are found with illness, SOD may help support the immune system in combating illnesses. Additionally, levels of SOD may be critical in determining one's susceptibility to infection.

- **SOD in patients with HIV.** A study reported in *Superoxide Dismutases: Recent Advances and Clinical Applications* discovered a reduced SOD effectiveness in patients with HIV despite an increase in their levels of internal SOD. The study also showed that HIV increases the level of ROS, specifically an abnormal accumulation of superoxide. In the study, 86 patients—46 of whom were HIV positive—were examined. All of the HIV-positive patients had higher levels of SOD, probably in response to the virus. However, a certain protein that plays a role in the progression of HIV was thought to interfere with the ability of the SOD to neutralize superoxide. As a result, excess levels of superoxide contributed to the damage of healthy cells and the proliferation of the virus.

• **SOD slows the spread of HIV in the body.** In another study in *Superoxide Dismutases: Recent Advances and Clinical Applications,* researchers added SOD to infected white blood cells from patients with HIV. The results showed that SOD slowed the spread of HIV through the infected cells. This is important for two reasons: First, white blood cells are a crucial part of the immune system. Because the HIV virus tends to "live" there, they can get killed off and jeopardize the health of the infected patient. Also, because white blood cells are a holding ground for the virus, it is thought that the virus's activity in those cells is responsible for its transmission. The study also found that superoxide was able to enhance cell-to-cell transmission of the virus. The reducing effect of SOD on superoxide seems to be not only on the level of HIV in the white blood cells, but also on the rate of transmission of the virus between cells.

• **SOD can slow the expression of HIV.** In another study reported in *Superoxide Dismutases: Recent Advances and Clinical Applications,* researchers tested the effect of SOD on HIV-infected macrophages. They found that SOD reduced the levels of the virus's core protein, an indicator of its presence in the cells. This suggests that SOD can prevent the expression of HIV to AIDS. Like other research, this study suggests the use of SOD in tandem with other drugs as a combination anti-viral therapy. It's important to note that in this study, the treatment was effective for up to 2 weeks after infection. Two weeks after infection, SOD had not effect on the levels of the core protein.

• **SOD can prevent T cell death.** A study reported in *Medical Hypotheses* focused on the relationship between apoptosis and AIDS. Researchers noted that oxidative stress plays a primary role in T cell apoptosis in patients with AIDS, mainly because AIDS patients have low levels of antioxidants such as SOD. Additionally, HIV-infected cells treated with antioxidants showed a lower rate of apoptosis. The researchers suggest that a complete anti-viral vaccine would include antioxidants such as SOD to help reduce T cell apoptosis.

Another study, reported in *Biochemical Pharmacology*, supported the theory that depletion of T cells in patients with HIV is aggravated by ROS. The resulting oxidant-antioxidant imbalance could be responsible for both the progression of HIV and the cellular destruction within the immune system.

- **SOD can boost the production of T cells.**
Certain levels of ROS are important because they
help the immune system destroy bacteria and
other microorganisms. However, these ROS may
be more detrimental in the case of age-related
immune deficiencies. A review in *Annals of
Clinical Laboratory Science* noted that antioxidants
such as SOD can counteract the damaging effects of ROS and other free radicals by actually
stimulating the production of T cells and other
important immune system components.

- **SOD can protect the lungs from damage.** A
study reported in the *Annals of the New York
Academy of Sciences* found that patients with acute
respiratory distress syndrome (ARDS) produced
high levels of interleukin-1 and neutrophils in response to the illness. Interleukins are specialized
proteins in the immune system that regulate the
production of blood cells. Neutrophils are special white blood cells that attack and destroy foreign invaders. One of the side effects of the
overproduction of these immune cells is lung
leak, or fluid in the lungs. The researchers found
that SOD reduced the amount of lung leak in
rats stimulated to have symptoms of ARDS.
Treatment also reduced the amount of other
free radicals. This study suggests that SOD can
help support the immune system by protecting
the lungs from excessive damage when combating ARDS.

- **SOD can enhance immunity.** A study in *Immunology Letters* examined the effect of oxygen free radicals on the immune systems of rabbits. In the study, researchers found that a higher-than-normal presence of free radicals affected the immune system both at cell-specific sites and throughout the bloodstream—an important point, since circulation is the transportation vehicle for the immune system. The presence of free radicals appears to contribute to the suppression of the immune system. SOD can counter the effects of ROS free radicals, thereby enhancing immune function.

Another study in *Immunitat und Infektion* reinforces the role of antioxidants in immunity. As part of the immune response, free radicals such as superoxide are produced, but these free radicals can cause tissue and immune system damage. Adding antioxidants through supplementation can be an important way to reduce the immune-damaging effects of these free radicals.

- **SOD can prevent damage to the immune system.** A study reported in *Proceedings of the Nutrition Society* found that ROS can damage the immune system in several ways. First, ROS can destroy immune system cells, thereby depleting the body's protective mechanism. Additionally, cell-to-cell communication is crucial to a well-functioning immune system, and ROS can interfere with that communication by damaging the cell membranes that are key in cell communication. This also can limit the effectiveness of an immune response. SOD can offset the detrimental effects of ROS to help maintain a healthy immune system.

• **SOD can normalize T cell activity in older people.** A study in the *American Journal of Clinical Nutrition* suggests that antioxidant protection is even more important in older people. Antioxidants are important in immune system function, including cellular communication and immune cell reproduction and integrity. In older people in particular, there tends to be a dysfunction in T cell activity. The effects of oxidation contribute to this problem, and antioxidants may help maintain and even enhance the function of the immune system in older people.

• **SOD can protect the immune system from environmental toxins.** The immune system is affected not only by viruses and disease but also by sunlight, cigarette smoke, and other environmental toxins. A review reported in the *Journal of Dairy Sciences* noted that a healthy immune system depends on the intake of micronutrients, which can act as antioxidants. Recent studies have found that supplementing with antioxidants can protect the immune system from environmental hazards and improve overall immune response. As an extremely powerful antioxidant, SOD may similarly protect the immune system.

Supplement Plan for Immune Support

From vitamin A to zinc, many nutrients are required to maintain a normal immune system. Immune support above and beyond what is obtained from a multiple-vitamin-and-mineral product is required for a healthy and effective immune response. The following nutrients (as well as the nutrients recommended for cancer in Chapter 3) can be used as part of an integrated treatment approach for immune support:

Foundation Nutrient
SOD/gliadin, 200–500 I.U.

Nutrients to Prevent Muscle/Tissue Loss
Undenatured Whey Protein
OKG (ornithine alpha ketoglutarate)
Branched Chain Amino Acids
Nucleotides
L-Glutamine

Antioxidant Support
Beta Glucans
Polyphenols

Coenzyme Q10
Nucleotides
High Immunoglobulin Whey Protein
L-lysine
L-Glutamine
Full multiple antioxidant formula, with emphasis on both water soluble and fat soluble antioxidants

Immunomodulating/Antimicrobial Herbs:
olive leaf, elderberry, scutellaria, andrographis, oregano, basil, reishi/shiitake & maitake mushrooms, tumeric, astragalus, cat's claw, isoflavones, modified citrus pectin

Mitochondrial/Energy Support
Coenzyme Q10
D-Ribose
L-Carnitine
MCT (medium chain triglycerides)
L-Glutamine

CHAPTER 6

SOD AND NEUROLOGICAL DISORDERS

We take it for granted that we'll be able to find our car keys, walk down the street, bathe, and put on our clothes. But if the brain isn't working properly, all the simple activities we take for granted—movement, memory, even speech—are affected. As we age, the likelihood of experiencing brain or neurological disorders increases dramatically, with often devastating consequences. The term "dementia," for example—often used to describe Alzheimer's disease—means "deprived of mind." It's an accurate enough description; neurological disorders strip their victims of basic and automatic mental and physical functions.

Neurological disorders are conditions that affect the brain and central nervous system, causing severe physical and mental dysfunction, including memory loss, speech difficulties, severe changes in judgment, and loss of motor function. Alzheimer's disease, Parkinson's disease, and amyotrophic lateral sclerosis (ALS), otherwise known as Lou Gehrig's disease, are some of the most common and most devastating neurological disorders. Other neurological disorders include multiple sclerosis, attention deficit hyperactivity disorder (ADHD), chronic fatigue syndrome, and depression. The inner complexities of the brain, immune system, and gastrointestinal tract and new nutritional approaches to these neurological diseases are fully described in my book *The Brain Wellness Plan.* Now there's more hope and a new nutritional player taking the spotlight: New research is finding that higher levels of SOD can slow the progress, and possibly even prevent the onset, of some of the most devastating forms of neurological disease.

Brainstorm: How the Brain Works

As complex as it is, the mechanisms by which the brain works aren't so different from those of other organs. To keep the brain healthy, a steady and ample supply of blood is crucial to carry oxygen and nutrients to the brain cells. The normal process of aging, however, interferes with brain function on a number of levels. The brain begins to lose capacity as early as the mid-40s, and even healthy adults may begin to lose up to 50% of the brain's function in the realm of memory and concentration. One reason is that occluded arteries and decreased circulation, typically related to aging, result in diminished blood flow to the brain.

Healthy brain function also depends on the consistent production and release of chemical messengers and neurotransmitters and the smooth flow of information. Optimal brain function requires flexible membranes that allow chemical messages to flow in and out. Again, aging is related to diminished brain function. As the brain ages, its membranes become rigid, thereby hampering the flow of information. Free radicals can also damage cell membranes.

Additionally, the brain requires ample antioxidant protection. Because it contains a great deal of fatty tissue, it's highly susceptible to free radical damage, which appears to be a common factor in diminished neurological function. For example, some studies show that the brains of Alzheimer's patients typically have 50% more free radical production. This is where antioxidants, such as SOD/ gliadin, can have a pronounced and beneficial effect on brain health.

Alzheimer's Disease

Alzheimer's disease is a progressive, neurodegenerative disease characterized primarily by memory loss. It can also include loss of speech capability and extreme changes in judgment and attitude. Early symptoms, which usually include forgetfulness and poor concentration, can be easily overlooked. And it's a huge problem: Nearly 4 million Americans suffer from Alzheimer's, and 10% of people over age 65 are thought to have some form of the disease. For people over age 85, that number skyrockets to nearly 50%. And as new scientific findings and improved medical capabilities continue to extend life expectancy rates and elderly populations grow, the number of people with neurological disorders continues to increase.

Alzheimer's appears to be caused by neurofibrillary tangles and plaque deposits in the brain's cells and blood vessels, which lead to cell damage and death. These alterations block certain normal brain functions, resulting in the symptoms common to Alzheimer's, such as memory loss, speech difficulties, and changes in judgment and attitude. Another factor is cerebrovascular beta-amyloidosis, or the depositing of starchlike proteins (amyloids) in the brain's circulatory system. Amyloids are toxic to the blood vessels in the brain, damaging cells and causing an increase in superoxide free radicals. Likewise, free radical imbalance can contribute to amyloid toxicity in a vicious cycle. New directions in how inflammation and the immune system's inflammatory cytokines and mitochondrial failure play critical roles in the development and further exacerbation of the disease is gaining increased attention within the medical community. Hence, the

Defining the Terms

Neurofibrillary tangles are neurons, or nerve cells, that have been damaged. The neuron looks like a fried egg, the yolk being the nucleus, with roots extending outward. These roots are called microtubules, and they are constructed like a railroad, with parallel tracks supported by cross members. They are responsible for carrying nutrients to and from the nerve cell. In the case of neurofibrillary tangles, the microtubules are collapsed and intertwined. This result has been associated with the presence of senile plaques and injury.

Senile plaques, commonly found in Alzheimer's patients, are typically groups of microglial cells—non-nerve cells in the central nervous system—clustered around amyloid deposits. Amyloid is composed mostly of amyloid beta protein and several other proteins. Researchers speculate that the brain's inability to break down excess amyloid proteins can lead to the buildup of senile plaques. These plaques can contribute to processes such as the degeneration of neurons and neurofibrillary tangles. There is a correlation between an increase in senile plaques and age, and an even stronger relationship between the presence of plaques and brain diseases such as Down's syndrome and Alzheimer's.

role of anti-inflammatory agents to calm and treat the disease. Additionally, more and more research is finding an association between low levels of SOD in the brain and increased probability of Alzheimer's. The hope is that SOD/gliadin can slow the progression and even prevent Alzheimer's.

Parkinson's Disease

Parkinson's disease is a progressive neurological disorder that affects the body's motor system. Identified by tremors—especially in the hands, arms, legs, and face—stiffness in the limbs, and imbalance, this disorder is a direct result of nerve cell damage due to aging, free radicals, and other factors. The damaged cells can no longer communicate properly with other cells, and motor ability becomes compromised. Parkinson's affects nearly 1.5 million Americans, almost all over the age of 30. Like most degenerative diseases, the causal factors can be traced to cellular damage. Because Parkinson's is associated with free radical damage, the hope is that SOD/gliadin can slow the onset and progression of the disease.

Amyotrophic Lateral Sclerosis

Amyotrophic lateral sclerosis (ALS), or Lou Gehrig's disease, is another progressive, neurodegenerative disease that affects the motor functioning of the individual. It is perhaps the deadliest of these diseases, usually allowing no more than 5 years between diagnosis and death. Like Parkinson's, ALS is caused by damaged neurons and the resulting inability to control voluntary movements. Manifestation of the disease may begin with poor circulation, tripping and falling, and difficulty speaking and swallowing. It ends with almost complete paralysis. As movement is increasingly restricted, the muscles atrophy and the body deteriorates. Ironically, though, the mind remains sharp and alert.

ALS affects nearly 20,000 Americans, with an estimated 5,000 new cases diagnosed every year. There is no cure and the treatments are symptomatic, attempting to make life a little easier for the victims. ALS has also been linked to heredity and defective chromosomes and enzymes, but the real cause is yet unknown. One hypothesis is that free radical damage in the cerebral cortex, brainstem, and spinal cord destroys nerves and neural functioning. Scientists have discovered a mutated version of SOD, one that is unable to combat free radicals, as a possible culprit in the destruction of nerve cells. Normal SOD in sufficient quantities seems to prevent ALS-related damage. It's likely, then, that SOD can prevent nerve degeneration and arrest or reduce the symptoms of ALS.

What the Studies Show

In recent years, science has sought to uncover the underlying and originating causes of neurological disorders. One prominent finding is that free radical damage appears to be one of the primary causes of these tragic diseases. Other studies have suggested that SOD can slow the progression, and even prevent the onset, of neurological disorders, including Alzheimer's, Parkinson's, and ALS.

One note: This research is new, and some studies have found that SOD may contribute to some of the physical characteristics leading up to these conditions, which further supports other conclusions that oxidative stress causes neurological disorders. As superoxide is dismutated by SOD, it produces hydroxyl (HO) and hydrogen peroxide (H_2O_2), two powerful ROS free radicals that can cause cellular and neuron damage. But SOD is also responsible for regulating the antioxidants glutathione and catalase, which dismutate these types of ROS. So, after reviewing all the science, the conclusion seems to be that more SOD is better and less SOD is detrimental. Following are some of the most conclusive studies pointing out SOD's effects on neurological disorders.

- **SOD protects the brain cells from damage.** A study in the *Journal of Neuroscience* confirmed SOD as a cell protector. In portions of the brain where circulation is restricted, cell death results in part from an increase in free radicals during the reduced blood flow. Neurological disorders occur because damaged or dying nerve and brain cells cannot function normally. This study found that additional SOD in the brain significantly reduced cell death in the presence of reduced circulation. Researchers suggested that supplementation with SOD can prevent unnecessary brain and nerve cell death especially in the case of restricted circulation.

A study in *Brain Research* showed an association between neurodegenerative diseases, ROS production, and glutamate neurotoxicity. We already know that ROS can cause some of the damage that leads to the diseases of the brain, and this study illuminates specific mechanisms. Researchers say that lower levels of SOD can lead to neuron damage in the brain through glutamate toxicity. Glutamate is an important and abundant neurotransmitter. Its general role is to create energy or excitement, as opposed to calming the brain. Like other systems in the body, a proper balance of components is required for optimal health. If too much glutamate exists, its stimulating effect can be destructive to the neurons. The study suggests that SOD can prevent excessive levels of glutamate, thereby offsetting neuron damage.

- **SOD levels are lower in Alzheimer's patients.** A study in *Alzheimer's Disease and Associated Disorders* explored the levels of SOD in patients with several types of neurological disorders. The study included 32 dementia patients (23 with Alzheimer's-type dementia, or DAT), 13 epilepsy patients, 12 Parkinson's patients, and 58 controls. The researchers found that lower levels of SOD were more evident in the dementia group and most pronounced in the DAT group. SOD activity in the DAT group was about 43% lower than in the control group. This suggests that diminished defense against ROS is largely responsible for the onset and progression of dementia, particularly Alzheimer's. Supplementing with SOD could prevent the beginning, and slow the progression, of neurological disorders, including Alzheimer's.

- **SOD levels are lower in patients with ALS.** A study in the *Journal of Neurochemistry* found that people with familial (inherited) ALS (FALS) carried a mutated version of SOD. As a result, the free radical fighting ability of SOD was reduced by up to 50% in the brain. Researchers suggest that the ineffectiveness of this mutated SOD could be what allows the levels of free radicals to increase, ultimately leading to neurological damage. Though not suggested by the study, the results imply that normal SOD could slow and prevent the damage that leads to neurological disorders such as ALS.

- **SOD can prevent neurological disorders.** A study reported in *Cellular and Molecular Neurobiology* suggests that oxidative stress can lead to neurological diseases specifically through the increase of ROS. Because the brain is so high in lipids and oxygen, the potential for oxidation (damage from oxygen-based free radicals) of those lipids is high. If ample antioxidants aren't present, oxidative stress can include the type of nerve damage that leads to neurodegenerative diseases such as Parkinson's and ALS. According to the researchers, therapeutic approaches that limit oxidative stress, such as supplementing with antioxidants, may be beneficial in the treatment of these neurological diseases.

- **SOD can prevent the development and progression of Parkinson's disease.** The mitochondria are the energy-producing units within the cells, including the brain cells. They are like cellular engines: If they don't work properly, the cell can neither function nor survive. A study in *Experimental Neurology* found that ROS can damage and impair the functioning of the mitochondria, leading to cell death, and that damage to brain cells from ROS appears to be one of the causes of Parkinson's. Researchers found that SOD protects the mitochondria from damaging ROS and that an overall balance of antioxidants, including SOD, can help prevent Parkinson's.

Another study, reported in the *Proceedings of*

the National Academy of Sciences of the United States of America, also noted that most of the ROS in cells is produced by the mitochondria. The study also found that when the genes in the body responsible for producing SOD are damaged, SOD production becomes abnormal, leading to cellular damage. This cellular damage could be the start of Parkinson's and other neurological disorders, including Alzheimer's and ALS.

A study in *Functioning Neurology* found that levels of superoxide were significantly higher in Parkinson's patients than in healthy test subjects. Further, they noted an increase in SOD activity as well. Researchers suggest that this increase in SOD is a "compensatory defensive reaction" to the higher levels of superoxide. However, this defensive burst soon wears off and is not enough to protect the brain from the continuous cycle of free radical damage. This study supports other findings that free radicals and oxidative stress play a key role in the development and progression of Parkinson's.

Another study, outlined in *Superoxide Dismutases: Recent Advances and Clinical Applications,* found a significant decrease in SOD activity in patients with Parkinson's compared to healthy controls. The study pointed to insufficient protection against ROS, and oxidative stress in general, as a possible cause or contributor to Parkinson's. Higher levels of SOD could prevent some of the damage leading to the disease.

• **SOD can prevent the development and progression of Alzheimer's disease.** A commentary by Benzi and Moretti in *Neurobiology of Aging* concluded that oxidative stress was at least a contributing factor in the onset of Alzheimer's. They stated that Alzheimer's favors conditions in the brain where ROS outnumbers antioxidants such as SOD. The decreased defense encourages the proliferation of free radicals, and the ensuing free radical damage creates a chain reaction affecting the mitochondria and the cell membrane, resulting in damaged and dying cells that can contribute to Alzheimer's. Researchers concluded that SOD protects the central nervous system and can help prevent Alzheimer's and other neurological disorders.

A study reported in *Brain Research* found that SOD may prevent the damage that leads to Alzheimer's. One characteristic of Alzheimer's is beta-amyloids in the brain's circulatory system. This study noted that SOD could prevent beta-amyloid toxicity, halting damage in both the blood vessels and the cells. Thus, SOD may play a role in preventing the damage that results in Alzheimer's.

Another study, reported in the *Journal of Molecular Neuroscience*, also concluded that beta-amyloids are responsible for creating oxidative stress, which damages brain cells. Specifically, they found that neurons in the brain activated a strong protective response, including an increase in the production of SOD, when beta-amyloid peptides were present. Eventually, the natural defenses were overwhelmed in this exaggerated experiment, and the neurons became damaged and died. The researchers noted that this oxidative damage plays a key role in the development of Alzheimer's. The study suggests SOD can prevent the oxidative damage that can result in Alzheimer's.

A study in the *Annals of New York Academy of Science* revealed that levels of SOD were significantly lower, by 25% to 35%, in the frontal cortex, hippocampus, and cerebellum areas of Alzheimer's brains than in those of controls. The hippocampus is the area of the brain that affects memory, and most scientists agree that the disease of Alzheimer's appears to affect primarily the hippocampus. Without adequate protection against free radicals, cellular and neurological damage that causes Alzheimer's can occur.

Another study, in *Superoxide Dismutases,* concurred that substances called alpha-beta-peptides contribute to the plaques that lead to damaged blood vessels in the brain, nerve cell death, and, ultimately, Alzheimer's. Alpha-beta-peptides result in an increase in free radicals, which leads to, among other things, damage to blood vessels and decreased oxygen flow. This study found that supplemental SOD resulted in less vascular constriction and less damage to blood vessel walls, thereby promoting circulation in the brain. Researchers suggest that the damage from alpha-beta-peptides can lead to greater levels of ROS, which, in turn, can destroy the mitochondria and the cell's ability to produce its own SOD. SOD protects against damage from alpha-beta-peptides.

A study in the *Journal of Neurological Sciences* compared levels of hydroxl radical (OH), a type of free radical, with SOD levels in the blood plasma of Alzheimer's patients and healthy controls. Researchers found that OH levels were significantly higher and SOD levels were significantly lower in Alzheimer's patients than in healthy subjects. This supports other findings that free radical damage plays a role in the onset and continuation of Alzheimer's. The study suggests that SOD can alleviate free radical damage and halt the onset or progression of Alzheimer's.

Supplement Plan for Neurological Disorders

Depending upon the illness, there are several approaches to take with a variety of important neuroprotective nutrients. Essentially, we again must abandon the single-magic-bullet approach and concentrate on the major components. The following nutrients can be used as part of an integrated treatment approach for neurological disorders:

Foundation Nutrient
SOD/gliadin, 200–500 I.U.

Neurotransmitter Support Nutrients
CDP choline
Acetyl-L-carnitine
Hyperzine A
Phosphatidylserine
Docosahexaeonic acid (DHA)
Standardized ginkgo biloba
Standardized rhodiola rosea (Rhodovin™)

Mitochondrial Resuscitator Nutrients
Coenzyme Q_{10}
Lipoic acid
Creatine
D-ribose (Ribocell™)

Antioxidant Support Nutrients
Complete multiple antioxidant formula
Glutathione modulators (N-acetyl-cysteine,
lipoic acid, selenium, and vitamin C)

Anti-inflammatory Nutrients
Standardized turmeric extract
Caffeic acid phenylester (CAPE)
Standardized nettle extract
Standardized white willow bark

Standardized devil's claw
Ursolic acid
Resveratrol
Standardized boswellia extract

CHAPTER 7

SOD and Vision

The primary function of our sensory organs is to protect us from harmful situations. Without touch we would be unable to differentiate between warm and scalding water. Without taste, a glass of spoiled milk would be just as satisfying as fresh milk even though it would contain harmful bacteria. If we were deaf, the horn of an oncoming car would never be heard. A gas leak in the kitchen would go unnoticed if we could not smell. To be blind means living in a maze of obstacles, sharp corners, and dead ends. Although these are minor examples, the importance of our senses cannot be understated. Without them reality doesn't exist.

Out of all the senses, sight is relied upon most to protect us from our environment, as well as to enjoy the beauty of the world. Without sight, this book becomes a meaningless pile of paper. Our eyes survey the world around us and guide us through life. These amazing organs immediately clarify objects as close as 6 inches and as far away as a mile. Without this ability to focus, we would have to own a pair of glasses for every possible viewing distance!

However, the gift of sight comes with a price. Light, the same energy that allows us to see, also contributes to the gradual degradation of eyesight. What is this correlation between light and eyesight, and how can antioxidants like superoxide dismutase help? In this chapter, we will explore the association between free radicals and eyesight, and how superoxide dismutase can help to delay vision loss.

To See How the Eye Sees: Basic Eye Physiology

The human eye is truly an amazing organ, capable of detecting an almost limitless variety of colors and images. The eye is a sphere of layered tissue, with each layer serving a particular function. The process of seeing begins when light passes through the iris, which is the colored portion of the eye. The iris acts as a self-contained light-metering system, constricting in brightly lit environments and dilating when it is dark. In this way, the amount of light entering the eye is not too much or too little.

After light enters the eye, the choroid and the retina process it. The choroid, which lies between the sclera and retina, serves to nourish the retina.

Blood flow through the choroid contains high levels of oxygen and nutrients necessary to maintain healthy cells. The retina is the inner layer of the eye and the most important for sight. Within the retina lie the retinal pigment epithelium and photoreceptor cells. It is this complex of pigmented tissue and photoreceptor cells that initiates the visual process. The retinal pigment epithelium is a group of cells that support the photoreceptor cells. They are named for the fact that they contain the pigment melanin, which decreases light scatter in the eye, much the same way sunglasses decrease excessive glare. There are two types of photoreceptor cells and each is named according to its shape. Rods are responsible for night vision. They do not distinguish colors, but are very sensitive to light, hence their role in night vision. Cones allow us to distinguish colors during the day or in well-lit environments. In each retina, there are approximately 100 million rod cells and 6 million cone cells. To understand how important eyesight is in our sensory arsenal, consider that the rod and cone cells in the eyes account for 70% of all the receptors in the body!

Within each photoreceptor cell is a complex of retinal, a vitamin A derivative, and the protein opsin. When light enters the eye through the iris, it strikes the retina and interacts with the retinal/opsin complex in every photoreceptor cell. Thus, an image is imprinted on the retina in a fashion similar to the way camera film captures a picture when the aperture is opened. From here, the imprinted image is transmitted to the brain via the optic nerve. In the brain, the information is organized and perceived. You could say that we "see" with our brain and that the eyes are merely a window to the brain. Just like any window, the eyes are subject to damage.

The Eye and the Free Radical Generation Equation

There are three distinguishing characteristics of the eye that predispose it to free radical production. First, the cells of the retina are high in unsaturated fatty acids. Second, because the choroid layer is highly vascular, the eye is exposed to high oxygen levels. Finally, light, particularly ultraviolet light, is a potent generator of free radicals. When these three ingredients are put together, an ideal environment for free radical production is created. Remember, free radicals love to attack lipid membranes, and what better place is there to do this than the lipid-rich cells of the eye? When free radicals attack lipids, the process is called lipid peroxidation, and it produces substances such as lipofuscin and malonaldehyde (MDA). These substances are toxic and damage healthy cells. In the eye, tissue regeneration is slow, so oxidative damage can accumulate. This means that accumulated tissue damage resulting from exposure to free radicals leads to progressive visual impairment. This impairment can manifest itself as various disorders, most notably as cataracts and age-related macular degeneration (AMD). It is ironic that light, the very thing we need to see, can potentially blind us as well.

Free Radicals and Cataracts

The clinical signs of cataracts is clouding of the lens of the eye sufficient to impair vision. More than two-thirds of people over the age of 60 will have a vision problem due to cataracts, with more than a million cataract operations performed each year in the United States. Although most cataracts develop slowly as a result of aging, they can strike at any age due to genetic predisposition, trauma to the eye, side effects associated with radiation therapy, and glucocorticoid medications. The theory that cataracts result from free radical damage is gaining acceptance. Cataractous lenses have been shown to have a decreased level of antioxidant protection compared to normal lenses. Additionally, cataractous lenses exhibit a higher level of malonaldehyde, the toxic by-product of lipid perioxidation. Further credence to the free radical theory comes from researchers who, experimenting with substances that generate free radicals in the lens, accelerated the onset of cataracts.

Cataracts may also be the result of cholesterol oxidation. As we saw in Chapter 4, free radicals easily oxidize cholesterol and contribute to atherosclerosis. How does this relate to the eye? A little-known fact is that the human lens contains the highest cholesterol content of any known biological membrane, and because of this, it is a prime target for free radical attack. In fact, cataractous lenses have been shown to contain quantifiable amounts of oxidized by-products of cholesterol. This oxidized cholesterol may account for the membrane damage associated with cataracts.

Free Radicals and Age-Related Macular Degeneration

Age-related macular degeneration, or AMD, is the major cause of gradual, painless visual loss in the elderly and second only to diabetes as the leading cause of blindness in the 45- to 64-year age group. Macular degeneration is the progressive loss of vision due to the physical disturbance of the center of the retina called the macula. It is here where visual acuity is at its greatest. With destruction of the macula, visual acuity is impaired. As the disease progresses, central vision is lost, leaving a black hole in the direct field of vision.

There are two types of AMD: dry and wet. Of the two, dry macular degeneration seems to be most associated with free radical activity. Because of this, we will focus our attention on this form of the disease. Dry macular degeneration begins with the accumulation of yellowish deposits, called drusen, in the macula. Over time, these drusen become larger and more numerous, and eventually cause the retina to atrophy and impair vision by interfering with photoreceptor function. The exact cause of dry AMD is still speculative, but once again, it is thought that free radicals may be the impetus behind the disease. More specifically, it is thought that the generation of free radicals is associated with exposure of the retina to light, particularly UV light.

Risk Factors for AMD

- Age over 50 years, especially over 65
- Caucasian race
- Accumulation of retinal deposits (drusen)
- Family history
- Cigarette smoking
- Arteriosclerosis
- Diet deficient in antioxidants
- Excessive exposure to bright light, especially UV light

SOD and Eye Protection

With the evidence accumulating that free radicals contribute to two of the leading causes of vision loss, it is logical to assume that the same elaborate antioxidant defense system found in other parts of the body is also found in the eye.

There is strong evidence suggesting that superoxide dismutase plays an integral role in the antioxidant protection of the eye. In the case of age-related macular degeneration, it is thought that a disproportionate amount of free radicals generate lipofuscin, the toxic by-product of lipid peroxidation. When exposed to light, lipofuscin perpetuates lipid and protein peroxidation, contributing to further retinal damage, which eventually progresses to AMD. Various levels of antioxidant enzymes, including superoxide dismutase, are depressed in the AMD patients, and the effects of lipofuscin were significantly reduced by the addition of this antioxidant enzyme. This suggests that free radicals and their by-products play an integral role in AMD, and the administration of antioxidants such as SOD can help delay the onset of this devastating disease. As we have seen with cataracts, free radicals may oxidize the cholesterol-rich environment of the lens and lead to clouding. The same as patients suffering from AMD, people with cataracts exhibit lower levels of antioxidants and higher concentrations of lipid by-products in the eye.

Studies have also shown that the levels of SOD in the adult eye are higher than in the fetus. Additionally, SOD levels increase simultaneously with the eyes' first opening after birth. This indicates that once the eyes are exposed to light, oxidative damage ensues, and that the damage is countered by increased production of superoxide dismutase. Although considerably more research has to be done in the field of antioxidants and their role in preserving eyesight, existing evidence strongly suggests that antioxidant enzymes like SOD play an integral role in preventing damage from free radicals and helps to preserve normal vision.

What the Studies Show

• **SOD may prevent cataracts.** Malonaldehyde is a by-product of lipid peroxidation and was shown to be higher in senile and complicated cataractous lenses than in normal human lenses. Superoxide dismutase activity of senile and cataractous lenses was significantly lower than in normal lenses. This study suggests that lipid peroxidation may be a contributing factor in cataract development and that superoxide dismutase may play a preventive role in the process.

• **Light causes free radical damage in the eye.** A study using fluorescent lighting conditions to mimic daylight found that light caused substantial lipid peroxidation, as evidenced by the formation of malonaldehyde. This study suggests that light that freely penetrates the eye can initiate oxidative damage, resulting in lipid peroxidation and the eventual formation of cataracts.

• **SOD plays important roles throughout the life cycle.** Superoxide dismutase activity was studied in the developing mouse retina. Both manganese SOD and copper-zinc SOD in the retina of mice older than 2 weeks were almost two times greater than in younger mice. This study suggests that SOD activity exists in the retina of the fetus and increases as its role in the protective system against free radicals increases in the maturing mouse.

• **SOD activity is greater in the adult vs. fetal retina.** An article presented in *Investigative Ophthalmology and Visual Science* compared the levels of copper-zinc and manganese SOD in human and fetal retinal epithelium cells. Researchers found that manganese SOD showed greater activity in the adult cells. Adult retinal epithelium cells were also more resistant to the effect of paraquat, a chemical that causes increased production of superoxide.

• **SOD protects the photoreceptor cells in the eye.** In another study, presented in *The Histochemical Journal,* researchers hypothesized that the photoreceptor cells might have a cellular protective potential that included manganese SOD induction because these cells can easily be impaired by light.

Supplement Plan for Vision

More than any other tissue in the body, the lens and retina are continually subjected to oxygen and intense light radiation. Light and oxygen exposure create free radicals. The eyes are constantly exposed and susceptible to the potent effects of free radical activity. It is important for the eyes to rely on sufficient nutritional antioxidant support to neutralize the effects of free radicals. Additionally, normal daily wear and strain on your eyes can lead to changes in your vision. Difficulty focusing, blurriness, and visual distortion are common changes that can affect the quality of your life. In light of our increased longevity and heightened chance of vision impairment, researchers are exploring the role certain nutrients may play in keeping eyes healthy and retarding eye damage. As with so many health conditions today, it seems that antioxidants are the key. The following nutrients can be used as part of an integrated treatment approach for vision support:

Foundation Nutrient
 SOD/gliadin, 200–500 I.U.

Supportive Eye Nutrients
 Taurine
 DHA (docosahexaenoic acid)
 Troxerutin
 Diosmin

Polyphenols (fruit, grape seed, pine bark, citrus bioflavonoids)

Lutein

Standardized billberry

Standardized eyebright

Standardized ginkgo biloba

Complete vitamin B complex formula

Complete antioxidant formula including coenzyme Q_{10}, lipoic acid, carotenoids, tocotrienols/tocopherols, selenium, and zinc

CHAPTER 8

SOD/GLIADIN

So why go through all the trouble of producing an oral supplement of superoxide dismutase? In light of recent discoveries that antioxidants play a role in disease, numerous studies have been conducted on dietary antioxidants such as vitamins E and C and carotenoids such as beta-carotene. Efforts to understand what role our natural antioxidant defense system plays in the disease process have also been undertaken, and SOD has attracted serious attention. In this book, we examined the correlation between SOD and disease prevention and treatment. Maybe you or someone you know is afflicted with cancer, heart disease, or some other malady. Because of the critical role SOD plays in the body, each chapter answered the very important question, "Why do we need superoxide dismutase?"

It seems that SOD is a very important antioxidant enzyme, so that incorporating it into a dietary regimen would be prudent. There's one problem. The use of SOD as a dietary supplement is limited because of its inability to be completely absorbed. When SOD is taken by mouth, it is largely broken down in the gastrointestinal tract, losing its biological activity. This is the reason that oral SOD supplements have been unsuccessful. To understand why it has been so difficult to produce an oral supplement of SOD, a brief lesson in enzymology is needed.

Enzymes: Life's Little Laborers

Without enzymes, most of the chemical reactions important for life would occur at a very slow rate, in fact too slow. The function of an enzyme is to act as a catalyst, a substance that speeds up the rate of a chemical reaction without being consumed by the reaction. For example, digestion is the chemical process of breaking food down into its component parts for absorption. Food itself doesn't spontaneously break down once it is eaten. Enzymes are required to assist in this process. Without them, a meal might take months or years to digest instead of a few hours. Like digestion, most chemical reactions in the body require enzymes.

Chemically, enzymes are proteins with a very specific shape, and it is this shape that determines the enzyme's function. For almost every chemical reaction in the body, there is a specific enzyme with a specific shape. Because of their specificity, enzymes can function only under very specific conditions of acid-alkaline balance (pH), temperature, and salinity. Stomach enzymes, for example, are activated by their acidic environment, whereas enzymes in the intestines are active only in alkaline solutions. If these conditions change, the enzyme distorts and loses its specific shape and function in a process known as denaturation. Like all enzymes, superoxide dismutase is active only under specific conditions in the body, and this explains why it has been so difficult to produce an oral SOD supplement. Exposing SOD to the acidic environment of the stomach denatures the antioxidant enzyme, effectively destroying its functionality.

It is estimated that as little as 0.0005% of SOD reaches the small intestines after ingestion, and the SOD that remains is unabsorbable! However, if we would somehow protect SOD as it passed through the digestive tract, it is possible that we could increase its absorption. The idea is simple: Use a substance that will coat the SOD enzyme in a protective layer, thereby preserving its functionality as it passes through the stomach. Once it has safely passed through the stomach, SOD is delivered into the small intestines in a bioactive form.

What the Studies Show

The following discussion of the efficacy of SOD/gliadin is adapted from *Molecular Mechanisms and Therapeutic Strategies Related to Superoxide Dismutase by the Oral Route* by Bernard Dugas, Ph.D. Dr. Dugas is a renowned expert in the research and scientific application of SOD and SOD/gliadin.

Recently, a team of French scientists developed the idea of new technology to encase a vegetarian source of SOD in a wheat-based polymer called gliadin. The true test for the new vegetarian SOD/gliadin complex lies in whether SOD will be protected from stomach acid and be delivered intact to the intestines. In a series of experiments, researchers demonstrated that the gliadin polymer protected SOD against stomach acids and digestive enzymes. Blood levels of SOD subsequently increased, which indicates that the antioxidant enzyme was effectively absorbed from the intestines. It is estimated that gliadin can increase the absorption of SOD by as much as 57%, and additional studies corroborate these findings. The effects of the SOD/gliadin complex are directly proportional to the amount absorbed—that is, the more consumed, the greater the effect—and this effect has been sustained for up to 12 hours after ingestion.

Other studies demonstrated increased absorption using the SOD/gliadin complex. Four groups of animals were fed either the SOD/gliadin complex, or saltwater. When SOD activity was measured,

Table 8-1. The effect of the SOD/gliadin complex on the production of the body's own SOD.

Rat's Diet	Units of SOD activity
Saltwater	585
SOD	585
Gliadin	722
SOD/gliadin complex	1,008

the SOD/gliadin group was shown to have generated the greatest increase in SOD activity. (See Table 8-1.) These results suggest that SOD/gliadin is better absorbed than SOD alone.

Additional studies compared the effects of oral vegetarian SOD/gliadin complex to those of an injectable form of SOD derived from bovine sources. SOD increased SOD activity in the liver with 0.03 milligram to 0.3 milligram per kilogram and SOD/gliadin increased activity with 0.003 milligram per kilogram. Therefore, results show that the SOD/gliadin complex promoted a tenfold SOD activity increase in the liver at the lower dosage.

SOD/Gliadin Complex and Immune Defense

The immune system is a complex organization of cells and chemicals that protect us from pathogens. Within this chemical arsenal, free radicals are generated to destroy bacteria and viruses. However,

Table 8-2. The effects of SOD on the anti-viral activity of AZT in HIV-infected cells.

SOD pretreatment	AZT (3 micrograms per mililiter	HIV-related protein (pg/ml)
No treatment	-	175±12
No treatment	+	99±8
Bovine copper/zinc SOD	_	125±4
Bovine copper/zinc SOD	+	92±4
SOD/gliadin	-	99±3
SOD/gliadin	+	8±1

Cells were preincubated for 24 hours with or without bovine copper/zinc SOD or SOD/gliadin biopolymers. They were cultured with or without AZT, and HIV-1 replication was evaluated by quantity of HIV-related protein.

once the threat has been removed, the same free radicals that afforded protection can also damage the body if not quenched. It has been shown that gliadin not only delivers a bioactive form of SOD to the intestines but also promotes its delivery across the intestinal wall and increases the activity of cellular SOD in various organs such as the liver. The latter is attributed to the increased absorption of SOD which liberates the body's own SOD, thus optimizing the overall antioxidant defense system.

Table 8-3. The effect of AZT and SOD on normal human cells and cells infected with HIV-1.

Preincubation	Superoxide stimulation	Superoxide anion (normal cells)	Superoxide anion (HIV cells)
Control	-	0.40±0.1	0.98±0.4
Control	+	1.75±0.2	3.25±0.5
Free bovine copper/ zinc SOD	-	0.25±0.1	0.52±0.2
Free bovine copper/ zinc SOD	+	0.99±0.1	1.55±0.4
Gliadin	-	0.95±0.2	1.70±0.3
Gliadin	+	2.50±0.3	4.70±0.2
SOD/gliadin	-	0.55±0.1	0.45±0.2
SOD/gliadin	+	0.90±0.2	0.55±0.1

Human cells chronically infected by HIV-2 were preincubated for 48 hours with or without free SOD or SOD/gliadin. The cells were analyzed for the ability to produce superoxide anions after stimulation. AZT promoted oxidative stress in normal human cells and in HIV-1 chronically infected cells. When cells were treated with SOD, production of superoxide anions was reduced, with SOD/gliadin giving the best results.

Animal studies have demonstrated that the oral administration of SOD/gliadin induces not only an increase in SOD activity in plasma and erythrocytes, but also an increase of SOD and other defense enzymes—catalase and glutathionine peroxydase—in the liver!

A study examining the effect of SOD/gliadin complex on the immune system showed a stimulation of the antioxidant defense system and an increase in other antioxidants in various tissues and especially in the liver. This inducing effect was transitory because at the end of the SOD/gliadin diet the tissue level of SOD activity returned to the baseline level. These results suggest that the immune system must be stimulated in order to obtain a maximum effect from SOD.

SOD/Gliadin Enhances the Effects of Anti-viral and Antibiotic Toxicities and Enhances the Medicines' Effects

SOD acts as a drug-detoxifying therapeutic, as well as an enhancer to the effects of some antimicrobial drugs. Scientists think that it achieves this by stimulating the natural antioxidant defenses of cells. Certain antimicrobial drugs, notably those used to treat AIDS and hepatitis C, act by causing oxidation reactions on the cellular level. Unfortunately, their use is often limited because of their toxicity. Most biological disorders associated with microbial infections, at least in part, are caused by cell inflammation and by an imbalance in oxidant and antioxidant molecules in the cells. Free radicals are associated with the inflammatory process, indicating a disturbance in the oxidant-antioxidant balance in the cells. In addition to the free radical onslaught brought on by inflammation, drugs such as the anti-HIV drug azidothymidine (AZT) exacerbate oxidative stress by promoting oxidation reactions in cells. Because of this, the use of certain drugs is limited because of their toxicity. If these drugs promote cellular toxicity because of oxidative stress, then SOD may delay this effect and allow a greater dosage or treatment duration during therapy. Superoxide dismutase may allow these drugs to work more effectively and for a longer period of time.

Superoxide dismutase's ability to decrease cellular toxicity associated with certain anti-viral drugs was demonstrated in human cells infected with HIV and treated with AZT. Cells incubated with SOD/gliadin complex boosted the effect of AZT, which in turn reduced the amount of HIV protein in infected cells. Proteins from the HIV virus can be used to determine the level of viral load in a cell; a lower load indicates a greater therapeutic effect. It seems that the SOD/gliadin complex in combination with AZT may reduce the viral load by making AZT more effective. When human cells infected with HIV were incubated with bovine or SOD/gliadin in a laboratory test and then cultured with or without AZT, SOD potentiated the anti-viral effect of AZT. (See Table 8-2.) AZT caused oxidative stress that, in turn, produced the superoxide anion, a negatively charged atom or group of atoms, which caused cellular toxicity. When the cells were prein-cubated with SOD, however, this effect was over-come. (See Table 8-3.)

Superoxide dismutase may also enhance the ef-fects of antiparasitic drugs. Interleukin-2 (IL-2) is a protein produced by cells to facilitate the immune response. Part of that response is to regulate the production of free radicals, such as superoxide, and nitric oxide. Both protect against infection, but too much of either molecule can be just as bad for the cells as too little. Excessive amounts of superoxide can combine with nitric oxide to form an extremely potent free radical—peroxynitrite. Peroxynitrite is very destructive and can lead to cellular toxicity and death. However, SOD, when combined with IL-2, enhances the activity of IL-2 and protects against toxicity associated with peroxynitrite synthesis.

Superoxide dismutase can reduce the produc-tion of the superoxide anion, which decreases per-oxynitrite synthesis and subsequent cell damage. Future combinations of IL-2 and SOD could be used not only to reinforce the therapeutic effect of IL-2 but also to limit its toxicity. Superoxide dismu-tase may enhance the effect of other immune pro-teins as well. For example, the immune protein alpha-interferon also plays a role in regulating the immune system, and levels of this protein rise during bouts of infection. Superoxide dismutase has been shown to increase the activity of alpha-interferon in cells infected with hepatitis C virus. In light of these results, combinations of drugs and the SOD/gliadin complex might be used to enhance the immune system while reducing the side effects associated with drug therapy.

The protective effect of SOD against drug-induced cell toxicity was also demonstrated in mice infected by the liver parasite *Leishmania donovani*.

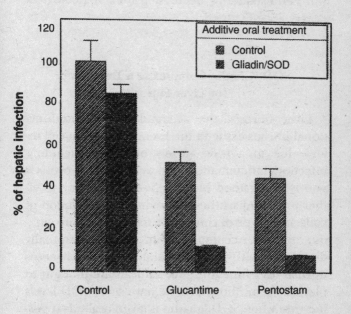

Figure 8-1. Effect of SOD on the activity of antiparasitic medicine. Three groups of five mice were infected with liver parasites and then given the antiparasitic medicines Glucantime® or Pentostam® for 2 weeks. Three other groups of five mice were given SOD/gliadin complex with Glucantime® or Pentostam®.

After mice were infected with parasites, they were then given one of the antiparasitic drugs Glucantime® or Pentostam® with or without SOD. One group received no antimicrobial drugs and served as a control. After 2 weeks, all the mice were killed and the parasites in their livers counted. SOD not only protected against liver toxicity but also increased the antimicrobial effect of Glucantime® and Pentostam® by decreasing their toxicological effects. (See Figure 8.1.)

SOD/Gliadin Complex as a Treatment for Liver Fibrosis

Liver fibrosis, the accumulation of nonfunctional fibrous tissue in the liver, results from cell injury due to a wide variety of agents including infection, inflammation, and toxic injury. Fibrosis is poorly understood but is believed to be due to either increased synthesis or reduced degradation of collagen, a type of connective tissue found throughout the body. Accumulated fibrous tissue eventually displaces healthy cells and ultimately compromises normal liver function. Free radicals are thought to play a role in fibrosis. As we have seen, SOD levels increase when SOD/gliadin is taken orally. Is it possible that increased SOD concentrations in the liver could protect against cell injury and resulting fibrosis? As noted before, when taken orally, SOD/

gliadin complex increased SOD production in the liver.

Two studies performed on animals demonstrate the effect of SOD on liver fibrosis. In the first experiment, mice were infected with liver parasites and then given SOD by injection for 7 weeks. One group of mice was sacrificed directly at the end of the dosing cycle, and a second was sacrificed 3 weeks later. In the second experiment, one group was force-fed SOD/gliadin, and another group received SOD by intramuscular injection. Both groups received SOD while being infected and for 16 weeks after. Results showed that the number of implanted parasites decreased and the development of fibrosis was controlled. SOD treatment improved the defense capacities of the liver against parasitic infection, and SOD/gliadin biopolymers taken orally up-regulated SOD production by the liver. Lastly, tissue studies measuring the density of fibrotic tissue caused by the liver parasites clearly indicated that SOD had a potent parasite-stopping and antifibrotic effect. Using subjects infected with liver parasites, SOD/gliadin complex decreased parasitic infection and controlled fibrosis. These results suggest that the SOD/gliadin complex can increase SOD activity in the liver and improve defense capacities of the liver against infection.

Neuroprotective Effect of
SOD/Gliadin Complex

Free radicals play an important role in aging and in the age-related degenerating processes that happen in the central nervous system. We know that excessive free radical production in the brain can cause cell death and can lead to cognitive dysfunction. Recent studies have demonstrated that SOD levels in the brain are correlated with neurodegeneration. In fact, some Alzheimer's patients have lower SOD activity in the cerebrospinal fluid, indicating that free radicals may contribute to dementia. Recent scientific studies have demonstrated that SOD probably influences the neurodegenerative processes by activating a cascade of the body's own antioxidative reactions. In turn, these reactions strengthen the cellular defense potential of certain cells in the central nervous system. These promising tests indicate a role for SOD/gliadin in the treatment of neurodegenerative processes, such as Alzheimer's disease, Parkinson's disease, and multiple sclerosis.

To study the effect of the SOD/gliadin complex on memory loss, subjects receiving radiation therapy for brain cancer are used, because this therapy has been shown to include aberrations in cognitive function similar to age-related memory loss. Using animals exposed to radiation, a decline in cognitive function was demonstrated by timing the animals' ability to avoid certain stimuli. The longer it took them to avoid the stimulus, the greater the neurological dysfunction. The SOD/gliadin complex reduced or delayed radiation-induced cognitive disturbances; that is, it increased the animals' ability to avoid the stimulus.

In this book, we examined the correlation between SOD and the diseases that are statistical leaders in morbidity and mortality. Maybe you are suffering or know somebody who is afflicted with cancer or heart disease or some other malady. Each chapter reinforces the assertion that free radicals play a significant role in the disease process and supplementing with SOD may reduce and even prevent certain diseases. Is SOD an important antioxidant enzyme? You be the judge.

REFERENCES

Introduction

Thomas JA. Oxidative stress, oxidant defense and dietary considerations. In: *Modern Nutrition in Health and Disease*. 8th ed. Philadelphia, Pa: Williams and Wilkins; 1994:501–10.

Melov S, Ravenscroft J, Malik S, Gill MS, Walker DW, Clayton PE, Wallace DC, Malfroy B, Doctrow SR, Lithgow GJ. Extension of life-span with superoxide dismutase/catalase mimetics. *Science*. 2000;289(5484):1567–69.

Huang TT, Carlson EJ, Gillespie AM, Shi Y, Epstein CJ. Ubiquitous overexpression of CuZn superoxide dismutase does not extend life span in mice. *J Gerontol A Biol Sci Med Sci*. 2000;55(1): B5–9.

De La Paz MA, Epstein DL. Effects of age on superoxide dismutase activity of human trabecular meshwork. *Invest Ophthalmol Vis Sci*. 1996; 37(9):1849–53.

Hussain S, Slikker W Jr, Ali SF. Age-related changes in

antioxidant enzymes, superoxide dismutase, catalase, glutathione peroxidase and glutathione in different regions of mouse brain. *Int J Dev Neurosci.* 1995;13(8):811–17.

Orr WC, Sohal RS. Extension of life-span by overexpression of superoxide dismutase and catalase in *Drosophila melanogaster. Science.* 1994;263 (5150): 1128–30.

Yen TC, King KL, Lee HC, Yeh SH, Wei YH. Age-dependent increase of mitochondrial DNA deletions together with lipid peroxides and superoxide dismutase in human live mitochondria. *Free Radic Biol Med.* 1994;16(2):207–14.

Liu J, Mori A. Age-associated changes in superoxide dismutase activity, thiobarbituric acid reactivity and reduced glutathione level in the brain and liver in senescence acceleterated mice: a comparison of ddY mice. *Mech Ageing Dev.* 1993; 71(1–2): 23–30.

De Lustig ES, Serra JA, Kohan S, Canziani GA, Famulari AL. Copper-zinc superoxide dismutase activity in red blood cells and serum in demented patients and in aging. *J Neurol Sci.* 1993;115(1): 18–25.

De Hann JB, Newman JD, Kola I. CU/Zn superoxide dismutase in mRNA and enzyme activity, and susceptibility to lipid peroxidation, increases with aging in murine brains. *Brain Res Mol Brain Res.* 1992;13(3):179–87.

Warner HR. Superoxide dismutase, aging and degenerative disease. *Free Radic Biol Med.* 1994;17(3): 249–58.

Kowald A, Kirkwood TB. A network theory of aging: the interactions of defective mitochondria, aberrant proteins, free radicals and scavengers in the aging process. *Mutat Res.* 1996;316(5–6): 209–36.

Niwa Y, Ishimoto K, Kanoh T. Induction of superoxide

dismutase in leukocytes by paraquat: correlation with age and possible predictor of longevity. *Blood.* 1990;76(4):835–41.

Nohl H. Involvement of free radicals in ageing: a consequence or cause of senescence. *Br Med Bull.* 1993;49(3):653–67.

Chapter 1

Bauerova K, et al. Role of reactive oxygen species in the etiopathogenesis of rheumatoid arthritis. *Gen Physiol Biophys.* Oct 1999; 18 Spec No:15–20.

Huber W, et al. Bioavailability of superoxide dismutase: implications for the anti-inflammatory mechanism of orgotein. *Agents Actons Suppl.* 1980; 7:185-95.

Laurindo IM, et al. Role of oxygen free radicals in the physiopathology of rheumatoid arthritis. *Rev Hosp Clin Fac Med São Paulo.* 1992;47(1): 38–45.

Tak PP, et al. Rheumatoid arthritis and p53: how oxidative stress might alter the course of inflammatory diseases. *Immunol Today.* 2000;21(2): 78–82.

Mapp PI, et al. Hypoxia, oxidative stress and rheumatoid arthritis. *Br Med Bull.* 1995;512: 419–36.

Heliovaara M, et al. Serum antioxidants and risk of rheumatoid arthritis. *Ann Rheum Dis.* 1994; 531: 51–53.

Niwa Y, et al. Effect of liposomal-encapsulated superoxide dismutase on active oxygen-related human disorders: a preliminary study. *Free Rad Res Comms.* 1985;12:137–53.

Corvo ML, et al. Intravenous administration of superoxide dismutase entrapped in long circulating liposomes. *Biochimica and Biophysica Acta.* 1999; 1419:325–34.

Gammer W, et al. Clinical comparison of orgotein and methylprednisolone acetate in the treatment of osteoarthritis of the knee joint. *Scand J Rheumatology.* 1984;13:108–12.

Taraza C, et al. Importance of reactive oxygen species in rheumatoid arthritis. *Rom J Intern Med.* Jan–Dec 1997;35(1–4):89–98.

Richard P, et al. Open clinical study of liposomal superoxide dismutase in severe rheumatoid arthritis. *Therapie.* Jul–Aug 1989;44(4):291–95.

McCord JM, et al. Superoxide and inflammation: a mechanism for the anti-inflammatory activity of superoxide dismutase. *Acta Physiol Scand Suppl.* 1980;492:25–30.

Chapter 2

Briscoe P, et al. Delivery of superoxide dismutase to pulmonary epithelium via pH-sensitive liposomes. *Am J Physiol.* 1995; 268 *(Lung Cell Mol Physiol* 12):L374–L380.

Montuschi P, et al. Increased 8-isoprostane, a marker of oxidative stress, in exhaled condensate of asthma patients. *Am J Respir Crit Care Med.* July 1999; 160(1):216–20.

Boljevic S, et al. Changes in free radicals and possibility of their correction in patients with bronchial asthma. *Vojnosanit Pregl.* Jan–Feb 1993; 50(1):3–18.

Comhair, SAA, et al. Rapid loss of superoxide dismutase activity during antigen-induced asthmatic response. *Lancet.* Feb 19, 2000;355:624.

Smith LJ, et al. Reduced superoxide dismutase in lung cells of patients with asthma. *Free Rad Biol Med.* 1997;22(7):1301–07.

DeBoer P, et al. Effects of endogenous superoxide anion and nitric oxide on cholinergic constriction of normal and hyperactive guinea pig airways. *Am J Respir Crit Care Med.* 1998;158: 1784–89.

Tekin D, et al. The antioxidant defense in asthma. *Asthma.* 2000;37(1):59–63.

Sanders SP, et al. Spontaneous oxygen radical production at sites of antigen challenge in allergic subjects. *Am J Respir Crit Care Med.* 1995; 151:1725–33.

Vachier I, et al. Increased oxygen species generation in blood monocytes of asthmatic patients. *Am Rev Respir Dis.* 1992;146:1161–66.

Misawa M, et al. Airway inflammation induced by xanthine/xanthine oxidase in guinea pigs. *Agent Actions.* 1993;38:19–26.

Chapter 3

Kogawa K, et al. Enhanced inhibition of experimental metastasis by the combination chemotherapy of Cu-Zn SOD and adriamycin. *Clini Exp Metastasis.* 1999;17:239–44.

Li JJ, et al. Inhibition of AP-1 and NF-KB by manganese-containing superoxide dismutase in human breast cancer cells. *FASEB J.* Dec 1998; 12:1713–23.

Miyachi Y, et al. Decreased skin superoxide dismutase activity by a single exposure of ultraviolet radiation is reduced by liposomal superoxide dismutase preteatment. *J Invest Dermatol.* 1987;89:111–12.

Sanchiz F, et al. Prevention of radioinduced cystitis by orgotein: a randomized study. *Anticancer Res.* 1996;16:2025–28.

Delanian S, et al. Successful treatment of radiation-induced fibrosis using liposomal Cu/Zn superoxide dismutase: clinical trial. *Radiother Oncol.* 1994; 32:12–20.

Martin-Mateo MC, et al. Assay for erythrocyte superoxide dismutase activity in patients with lung cancer and effects on pollution and smoke trace elements. *Biol Trace Element Res.* 1997;60:215–26.

Akashi, M, et al. Anti-cancer agent OK432 induces manganese superoxide dismutase in human granulocytes. *Int J Cancer.* 1996;68:384–90.

Wei LK, et al. The clinical and laboratory studies of superoxide dismutase activity in the human whole blood with early gastric cancer. *Free Rad Res Comms.* 1991;12–13:759–60.

Puscas I, et al. Erythrocyte superoxide dismutase activity in patients with digestive cancer: adjuvant diagnosis test. *Cancer Letters.* 1999;143:95–98.

Nimrod A, et al. The use of superoxide dismutase inhalation prevents lung fibrosis, but does not interfere with the anti-tumor effect in bleomycin-treated mice. In: Edeas MA. *Superoxide Dismutases: Recent Advances and Clinical Applications.* Editions Mel, Paris, 1999:196–99.

Chapter 4

Vaille A, Jadot G. Normolipidaemic activity of liposomal-encapsulated superoxide dismutase in rats. *Free Rad Res Comms.* 1990;11:4–5, 241–50.

Kobayashi A, et al. Oxygen-derived free radicals related injury in the heart during ischemia and reperfusion. *Jpn Circ J.* 1989;53:1122–31.

Bando K, et al. Twelve-hour cardiopulmonary preservation using donor care cooling, leukocyte depletion and liposomal superoxide dismutase. *J Heart Lung Transplant.* 1991;10:304–9.

Tatebe S. Myocardial protection of neonatal heart by cardioplegic solution with recombinant human superoxide dismutase. *Ann Thorac Surg.* 1992; 54:1, 124–29.

Nishikawa Y. The effect of superoxide dismutase and catalase on myocardial reperfusion injury in the isolated rat heart. *Jpn J Surg.* 1991;21:4, 423–32.

Pisarenko OI. Human recombinant extracellular superoxide dismutase type C improves cardioplegic protection against ischemia/reperfusion injury in isolated rat heart. *J Cardiovasc Pharmacol.* 1994; 24:4, 655–63.

Yen HC. Manganese superoxide dismutase protects mitochondrial complex I against adriamycin-induced cardiomyopathy in transgenic mice. *Arch Biochem Biophys.* 1999;362:1, 59–66.

Melov S. A novel neurological phenotype in mice lacking mitochondrial manganese superoxide dismutase. *Nat Genet.* 1998;18:2, 159–63.

Kinscherf R. Introduction of mitochondrial manganese superoxide dismutase in macrophages by oxidized LDL: its relevance in atherosclerosis of humans and heritable hyperlipidemic rabbits. *FASEB J.* 1997;11:14, 1317–28.

Xu MF. Effects of superoxide dismutase on ischemic reperfusion injury in isolated working heart and cultured myocardial cells of rats. *Chung Ku Yao Li Hsueh Pao.* 1990;11:4, 324–28.

Chapter 5

Umeki S, et al. Concentrations of superoxide dismutase and superoxide anion in blood of patients with respiratory infections and compromised immune systems. *Clin Chem.* 1987;33(12):2230–33.

Edeas MA, et al. High increase in Cu, ZN and Mn superoxide dismutase levels in plasma of individuals infected with human immunodeficiency virus type 1 is associated with high increase of TGF-ß1. In: Edeas MA. *Superoxide Dismutases: Recent Advances and Clinical Applications.* Editions Mel, Paris, 1999:162–67.

Edeas MA, et al. Effects of superoxide dismutase on HIV-1 replication. In: Edeas MA. *Superoxide Dismutases: Recent Advances and Clinical Applications.* Editions Mel, Paris, 1999:211–23.

Romero-Alvira D, et al. The keys of oxidative stress in acquired immune deficiency syndrome apoptosis. *Med Hypotheses.* 1998;51:169–73.

Baier-Bitterlich G, et al. Chronic immune stimulation, oxidative stress, and apoptosis in HIV infection. *Biochem Pharmacol.* 1997;53(6):755–63.

Knight JA. Review: Free radicals, antioxidants, and the immune system. *Ann Clin Lab Sci.* 2000; 30(2): 145–58.

Hybertson BM, et al. Phagocytes and acute lung injury: dual roles for interleukin-1. *Ann N Y Acad Sci.* 1997;832:266–73.

Koner BC, et al. Effects of in-vivo generation of oxygen free radicals on immune responsiveness in rabbits. *Immunol Lett.* 1997;59(3):127–31.

Biesalski HK, et al. Antioxidants in nutrition and their importance in the anti-/oxidative balance in the immune system. *Immun Infekt.* 1995;23(5):1166–73.

Hughes DA. Effects of dietary antioxidants on the immune function of middle-aged adults. *Proc Nutr Soc.* 1999;58(1):79–84.

Meydani SN, et al. Antioxidants and immune response in aged persons: overview of present evidence. *Am J Clin Nutr.* 1995;62(6 Suppl): 1462S–76S.

Hoffmann-LaRoche Inc. Physiological role of antioxidants in the immune system. *J Dairy Sci.* 1993; 76(9):2789–94.

Chapter 6

Fujimura M, et al. The cytosolic antioxidant copper/zinc–superoxide dismutase prevents the early release of mitochondrial cytochrome c in ischemic brain after transient focal cerebral ischemia in mice. *J Neurosci.* April 15, 2000; 20(8):2817–24.

Li Y, et al. Reduced mitochondrial manganese–superoxide dismutase activity exacerbates glutamate toxicity in cultured mouse cortical neurons. *Brain Res.* Dec 14, 1998;814 (1–2): 164–70.

De Deyn PP, et al. Superoxide dismutase activity in cerebrospinal fluid of patients with dementia and some other neurological disorders. *Alzheimer's Dis and Associated Disord.* 1998;12(1): 26–32.

Browne SE, et al. Metabolic dysfunction in familial, but not sporadic, amyotrophic lateral sclerosis. *J Neurochem.* 1998;71(1):281–87.

Facchinetti F, et al. Free radicals as mediators of neuronal injury. *Cell Mol Neurobiol.* 1998;18(6): 667–82.

Merad-Saidoune M, et al. Overproduction of Cu/Zn–superoxide dismutase or Bcl-2 prevents the brain mitochondrial respiratory dysfunction induced by glutathione depletion. *Exp Neurol.* Aug 1999;158(2):428–36.

Melov S, et al. Mitochondrial disease in superoxide dismutase 2 mutant mice. *Proc Natl Acad Sci USA*. Feb 2, 1999;96(3):846–51.

Ilic TV, et al. Oxidative stress indicators are elevated in de novo Parkinson's disease patients. *Func Neurol.* 1999;14(3):141–47.

Rapuzzi S, et al. Total superoxide dismutase (SOD) activity in human platelets during normal aging and in neurodegenerative disorders. In: Edeas MA. *Superoxide Dismutases: Recent Advances and Clinical Applications*. Editions Mel, Paris, 1999; 112–15.

Benzi G, Moretti A. Are reactive oxygen species involved in Alzheimer's disease? *Neurobiol Aging*. 1995;16(4):661–74.

Suo Z, et al. Superoxide free radical and intracellular calcium mediate Aß-42 induced endothelial toxicity. *Brain Res*. 1997;762:144–52.

Yatin SM, et al. Temporal relations among amyloid ß-peptide-induced free-radical oxidative stress, neuronal toxicity, and neuronal defensive responses. *J Mol Neurosci*. 1999;11:183–97.

Richardson JS. Free radicals in the genesis of Alzheimer's disease. *Ann N Y Acad Sci*. Sep 23, 1993;695:73–76.

Price JM, et al. The protective effect of SOD on vascular endothelium dysfunction induced by the Alzheimer's peptide. In: Edeas MA, ed. *Superoxide Dismutases: Recent Advances and Clinical Applications*. Editions Mel, Paris, 1999:89–94.

Ihara Y, et al. Free radicals and superoxide dismutase in blood of patients with Alzheimer's disease and vascular dementia. *J Neurol Sci*. 1997; 153:76–81.

Chapter 7

Oliver P, et al. Mitochondrial superoxide dismutase in mature and developing human retinal pigment epithelium. *Invest Ophthalmol Vis Sci.* 1992;33; 1909–18.

Behndig A, et al. Superoxide dismutase isoenzymes in the human eye. *Invest Ophthalmol Vis Sci.* 1998; 39:471–75.

Karlsson K, et al. Turnover of extracellular superoxide dismutase in tissues. *Lab Invest.* 1994;70: 705–10.

Yamamoto M, et al. Changes in manganese superoxide dismutase expression after exposure to intense light. *Histochem J.* 1999;31:81–87.

De La Paz M, et al. Effects of age on superoxide dismutase activity of human trabecular meshwork. *Invest Ophthalmol Vis Sci.* 1996;37: 1849– 53.

Marta S, et al. Free radical mediated effects in reperfusion injury: a histological study with superoxide dismutase and EGB 761 in rat retina. *Ophthalmic Res.* 1991;23:225–34.

Yamamoto F, et al. Effects of intravenous superoxide dismutase and catalase on electroretinogram in the cat postischemic retina. *Ophthalmic Res.* 1994; 26:163–68.

Horton JC. Disorders of the eye. In: *Principles of Internal Medicine.* 14th ed. New York: McGraw-Hill; 1998: 159–72.

Campbell NA. *Biology.* 3rd ed. New York: Benjamin/ Cummings Publishing; 1993:1020–26.

Yamashita H, Horie K, Yamamoto T, Katagirl H, Asano T, Hirano T, Nagano T, Oka Y. Super-oxide dismutase in developing mouse retina. *Jpn J Ophthalmol.* 1994;38:148–61.

Desrochers PE, Hoffert R. Superoxide dismutase provides protection against the hyperoxia in the retina of the rainbow trout *(Salmo gairdneri)*. *Comp Biochem Physiol*. 1983;76B(2):241–47.

Newsome DA, Dobard EP, Liles MR, Oliver PD. Human retinal pigment epithelium contains two distinct species of superoxide dismutase. *Invest Ophthalmol Vis Sci*. 1990;31(12):2508–13.

Varma SD, Srivastava VK, Richards RD. Photoperoxidation in lens and cataract formation: preventive role of superoxide dismutase, catalase and vitamin C. *Ophthalmic Res*. 1982; 14(3):167–75.

Lian H, Li S, Cao X, Pan S, Liang S. Malonaldehyde, superoxide dismutase and human cataract. *Yen Ko Hsueh Pao*. 1993; 9(4):186–89.

Chapter 8

Thomas JA. Oxidative stress, oxidant defense and dietary considerations. In: *Modern Nutrition in Health and Disease*. 8th ed. Philadelphia, Pa: Williams and Wilkins; 1994:501–10.

Melov S, Ravenscroft J, Malik S, Gil MS, Walker DW, Clayton PE, Wallace DC, Malfroy B, Doctrow SR, Lithgow GJ. Extension of life-span with superoxide dismutase/catalase mimetics. *Science*. 2000; 289(5484):1567–69.

Huang TT, Carlson EJ, Gillespie AM, Shi Y, Epstein CJ. Ubiquitous overexpression of CuZn superoxide dismutase does not extend life span in mice. *J Geronotol A Biol Sci Med Sci*. 2000;55(1): B5–9.

De La Paz MA, et al. Effects of age on superoxide dismutase activity in human trabecular meshwork. *Invest Ophthalmol Vis Sci*. 1996; 37:1849– 53.

Hussain S, Slikker W Jr, Ali SF. Age-related changes in antioxidant enzymes, superoxide dismutase, catalase, glutathione peroxidase and glutathione in different regions of mouse brain. *Int J Dev Neurosci.* 1995;13(8):811–17.

Orr WC, Sohal RS. Extension of life span by overexpression of superoxide dismutase and catalase in *Drosophila melanogaster. Science.* 1994; 263(5150): 1128–30.

Yen TC, King KL, Lee HC, Yeh SH, Wei YH. Age-dependent increase of mitochondrial DNA deletions together with lipid peroxides and superoxide dismutase in human live mitochondria. *Free Radic Biol Med.* 1994;16(2):207–14.

Liu J, Mori A. Age-associated changes in superoxide dismutase activity, thiobarbituric acid reactivity and reduced glutathione level in the brain and liver in senescence accelerated mice: a comparison of ddY mice. *Mech Ageing Dev.* 1993; 71(1–2): 23–30.

De Lustig ES, Serra JA, Kohan S, Canziani GA, Famulari AL. Copper-zinc superoxide dismutase activity in red blood cells and serum in demented patients and in aging. *J Neurol Sci.* 1993;115(1): 18–25.

De Hann JB, Newman JD, Kola I. Cu/Zn superoxide dismutase in mRNA and enzyme activity, and susceptibility to lipid peroxidation, increases with aging in murine brains. *Brain Res Mol Res.* 1992; 13(3):179–87.

Warner HR. Superoxide dismutase, aging and degenerative disease. *Free Radic Biol Med.* 1994; 17(3): 249–58.

Kowald A, Kirkwood TB. A network theory of aging: the interactions of defective mitochondria, aberrant proteins, free radicals and scavengers in the aging process. *Mutat Res.* 1996; 316(5–6): 209–36.

Niwa Y, Ishimoto K, Kanoh T. Induction of superoxide

dismutase in leukocytes by paraquat: correlation with age and possible predictor of longevity. *Blood.* 1990;76(4):835–41.

Nohl H. Involvement of free radicals in ageing: a consequence of cause of senescence. *Br Med Bull.* 1993;49(3):653–67.

INDEX